Clinical Melioidosis

Melioidosis is an endemic tropical disease and is fast becoming an emerging global concern. Its clinical mimicry with several other common diseases has made its diagnosis and treatment difficult. This book identifies a gap in the literature and represents the management and diagnosis of this fatal but potentially curable disease. It also provides detailed coverage of its history, epidemiology, the latency of the agent, pathogenesis, manifestations, clinical clues for detection, microbiological diagnosis, treatment, prevention, and environmental aspects. This book is for clinicians, infectious disease specialists, microbiologists, and public health professionals in countries where melioidosis is endemic.

Key Features:

- Provides practical guidance on clinical diagnosis, management, and prevention of melioidosis.
- Features high-quality radiological and clinical photographs for clinicians and professionals.
- Explores the latest techniques and advancements in laboratory diagnosis.

Clinical Melioidosis
A Practical Guide to Diagnosis and Management

Edited by

Prasanta Raghab Mohapatra

MD, FAMS, FRCP (London), FRCP (Glasg), FACP, FCCP,
FIDSA, ATSF, FICS, FICP, FAPSR
Dean (Academic), All India Institute of Medical Sciences.
Professor and Head, Department of Pulmonary Medicine &
Critical Care, AIIMS, Bhubaneswar, India

Foreword By

Bart Currie

Professor in Medicine,
Menzies School of Health Research, Charles Darwin University
and Royal Darwin Hospital, Darwin, Northern Territory, Australia

Ashutosh Biswas

Executive Director,
All India Institute of Medical Sciences, Bhubaneswar, India

CRC Press
Taylor & Francis Group
Boca Raton London New York

CRC Press is an imprint of the
Taylor & Francis Group, an **informa** business

First edition published 2023
by CRC Press
6000 Broken Sound Parkway NW, Suite 300, Boca Raton, FL 33487-2742

and by CRC Press
4 Park Square, Milton Park, Abingdon, Oxon, OX14 4RN

CRC Press is an imprint of Taylor & Francis Group, LLC

ISBN: 978-1-032-34828-5 (hbk)
ISBN: 978-1-032-34827-8 (pbk)
ISBN: 978-1-003-32401-0 (ebk)

DOI: 10.1201/9781003324010

Typeset in Times
by KnowledgeWorks Global Ltd.

To my heavenly Parents, wife Prof. Baijayanti, and children Ritik and Vaidehi, whose accomplishments have been a source of my pride and joy.

Contents

Foreword

Melioidosis has historically been considered a fascinating but rare tropical disease from southeast Asia and northern Australia. The last decade has seen an expansion of the global map of endemic melioidosis to include an increasing number of countries in Asia, Africa, and the Americas. Notable has been the recent exponential increase in publications of case reports and case series from India and Sri Lanka. Modelling estimated that India might account for more than 50,000 of the 165,000 cases of melioidosis predicted globally for 2015 and more than 30,000 of the predicted 89,000 global fatalities from melioidosis. Given the complexities of diagnosing and treating melioidosis, these estimates are very concerning and make this book very timely and valuable for clinicians and laboratory and public health staff—from those who are first hearing and wondering about this enigmatic 'great mimicker' to those experienced with its manifestations, diagnosis, and therapy but seeking more information and up-to-date advice.

Laboratory diagnostic technologies and genomic advances are revolutionizing the capacity for diagnostic and epidemiological answers at both individual patient and population levels. Nevertheless, access to such resources remains grossly inequitable for much of the world and this includes South Asia. The vast clinical diversity of melioidosis and the complexities of laboratory diagnosis and treatment make it truly a sentinel disease for highlighting the continuing global disparities in access to and provision of healthcare. This book shows us what is possible for diagnosis and therapy of melioidosis and to what we all as nations and a global community must continue to aspire.

Bart Currie
Professor in Medicine
Menzies School of Health Research, Charles Darwin University
and Royal Darwin Hospital, Darwin, Northern Territory, Australia

Foreword

Melioidosis is an infectious disease in tropical countries with varied clinical manifestations, a great mimicker, and a hidden killer. This book identifies a gap in the literature and represents the management and diagnosis of this fatal but curable disease. It provides detailed coverage of its history, epidemiology, the latency of the agent, pathogenesis, manifestations, clinical clues for detection, microbiological diagnosis, treatment, prevention, and environmental aspects. This book is the first clinical book on melioidosis that discusses clinical diagnosis and management from the clinician's perspective. The book is published at a pivotal moment when melioidosis is becoming a threat even in the non-endemic areas. The clinicians, post-graduates, and researchers working in melioidosis-endemic regions recognize a need for such a publication.

Faculty have devoted their valuable time to their contributions. They endeavoured to provide a comprehensive insight into the disease by discussing the various aspects of clinical melioidosis, from presentation to prevention, in this book.

The difficulties of diagnosing melioidosis and treating it are very concerning, and this book will be valuable for clinicians, laboratory, and public health staff—from those who are first hearing and wondering about this enigmatic disease to those who experienced its manifestations, diagnosis, and therapy, but are seeking more information and up-to-date advice.

My best wishes and congratulations to the multidisciplinary panel of 22 faculty members of All India Institute of Medical Sciences, Bhubaneswar, Prof. DAB Dance of the UK, and Bart Currie of Australia, who contributed to creating this important and first clinical book on melioidosis. I feel proud to see my team of faculty members who have made significant contributions to increasing awareness and better management of such fatal infectious cases in tropical countries.

Prof. Ashutosh Biswas
Executive Director
All India Institute of Medical Sciences, Bhubaneswar, India

Preface

Throughout human history, infectious diseases have been the leading cause of human morbidity and mortality. There has been an increase in infectious diseases over the last 25 years. I have experienced reasonable numbers of patients clinically mimicking an aggressive type of tuberculosis (never proving to have tuberculosis), becoming very sick in days. Many had died of sepsis and multi-organ abscesses without a specific microbial diagnosis.

There are likely many undiagnosed and unreported cases in tropical countries where endemic melioidosis is rarely clinically suspected. A predictive modeling study of the global distribution of melioidosis by Limmathurotsakul and colleagues estimated 165,000 melioidosis cases and 89,000 deaths worldwide in 2015. Melioidosis has been 'severely under-reported in 45 countries in which it is known to be endemic' and 'probably endemic in a further 34 countries that have never reported the disease'.

On the other hand, early intensified case detection and proper case management can decrease the case fatality rate of melioidosis from 90% to less than 15%, as reported in Australia. Key efforts remained to increase awareness for clinicians and public health workers by educating them to remain aware of potential clinical presentations and outbreaks.

We have gained a new perspective over the years and learned, with the support of microbiologists, that the disease increased after strong cyclonic weather events; all these facts incited us to develop the concept of this book, *Clinical Melioidosis: A Practical Guide to Diagnosis and Management*. This is probably the only clinical book that discusses from basics to bedside for every clinician, researcher, and healthcare professional. This book focuses on the integrated, holistic, essential clinical diagnosis and management of the dreaded disease in addition to introductory chapters. This book has elucidated treatment methods and best practices. We aim to fill the gaps in the knowledge of the physicians and surgeons on the clinical aspects of the disease, a great mimicker of many diseases. As an infectious disease, it is fully treatable with appropriate early management and preventable with due precautions. The information presented in this book is not only an up-to-date review of melioidosis, but also provides a comprehensive clinical insight into each aspect.

We published papers and review articles, including the latest in *Lancet Regional Health*, 'Burden of melioidosis in India and South Asia: Challenges and ways forward', to increase awareness and prevention of the disease. Investment in research for melioidosis lags far behind other neglected and emerging tropical diseases. There have been significant gaps in understanding this enigmatic disease's molecular epidemiology, transmission, and unpredictable behavior.

All the authors have devoted their valuable time to bring about their contributions. With the support of all the contributing authors, we discussed the various aspect of clinical melioidosis, from presentation to prevention, in this book.

This compilation has brought together a multi-disciplinary clinical faculty of authors who have summarized the updated literature to produce a complete clinical book on the subject.

I thank all the authors and their departments for contributing with devotion to this book. We express our gratitude and appreciation to the staff members of CRC Press (Taylor & Francis Group) for bringing this book to life. The CRC press brought the neglected tropical disease to the scientific societies through its publishing.

Prasanta R Mohapatra

Acknowledgement

I want to express my gratitude to the faculty and residents of the All India Institute of Medical Science, who made me realize the need for a clinical book on melioidosis.

My special thanks to Professor DAB Dance, University of Oxford, UK, and Professor Bart Currie, Director, Tropical and Emerging Infectious Diseases, for their contributions and constant encouragement.

I am thankful to all the contributors and faculty who supported me largely by giving constant encouragement and input. I am grateful to all the authors for giving their valuable time despite their busy schedules. I am appreciative to the support of all the faculty, staff, nursing officers, and faculty of my department for this work. My notable thanks to Dr. Biswanath Behera, Assistant Professor, Dermatology, AIIMS, Bhubaneswar, for their contribution to skin photography.

I express my immense gratitude to Prof. Pinaki Panigrahi, Director of International Microbiome Research, Georgetown University, Washington, DC, and Dr. Ena Mahapatra, Rush University, Chicago, USA. I further recognise Prof. Shyam Biswal, Johns Hopkins Bloomberg School of Public Health, USA, Dr. Suman Kumar Das, Stepping Hill Hospital, Manchester, UK, and Dr. Satya Mohan Mishra, John H. Stroger Jr. Hospital of Cook County, Chicago, USA, for their encouragement and needful input for this book.

I have no words to express my appreciation for my wife Dr. Baijayanti, son Ritik, and daughter Vaidehi, who have immensely cooperated with me throughout the process.

I am grateful to CRC Press for accepting my proposal to publish this book for a great cause. My sincere thanks to Ms. Shivangi Pramanik, Senior Editor-Medicine, and Himani Dwivedi, Editorial Assistant, for all their cooperation and positive efforts. I extend my thanks to all those who helped me bring this book to fruition.

Prasanta R Mohapatra

About the Editor

Prasanta Raghab Mohapatra
MD, FAMS, FRCP (London), FRCP (Glasg), FIDSA, FACP, FCCP, ATSF, FICS, FICP, FAPSR

Dr. Mohapatra is The Dean (Academic) of All India Institute of Medical Sciences, Bhubaneswar and has been Professor and Head of the Department of Pulmonary Medicine and Critical Care at All India Institute of Medical Sciences, Bhubaneswar, since April 2013. He is a Fellow of the Infectious Disease Society of America (IDSA) as well as an active Fellow of 16 scientific societies, including the Fellow of National Academy of Medical Sciences, the Royal College of Physicians of London and Glasgow, and a Fellow of the American College of Physicians, Fellow of the American College of Physicians, American College of Chest Physicians, and American Thoracic Society.

He has over 270 publications to his credit. He has been the Principal investigator of many projects and worked as Regional Editor for *Lancet Respiratory Medicine* (2015–2017). He was a committee member of several national guidelines, including the National Guideline Committee on Adult Vaccination 2019–2021.

He is the founder faculty of his department and a key clinical person for melioidosis work in his institution. He handled many cases from his setup and was instrumental in the melioidosis awareness services. During COVID-19, he has served as Chief Clinical Expert to the state and central team members in Maharashtra and Odisha. His leadership has focused on improving quality and delivering value to patient care, research, and teaching.

Contributors

Rama Chandra Barik
Department of Cardiology
All India Institute of Medical Sciences
Bhubaneswar, India

Bijayini Behera
Department of Microbiology
All India Institute of Medical Sciences
Bhubaneswar, India

Sanjeev Kumar Bhoi
Department of Neurology
All India Institute of Medical Sciences
Bhubaneswar, India

Sourin Bhuniya
Department of Pulmonary Medicine
    and Critical Care
All India Institute of Medical Sciences
Bhubaneswar, India

David AB Dance
Centre for Tropical Medicine & Global
    Health
University of Oxford
Oxford, United Kingdom
and
London School of Hygiene and Tropical
    Medicine
University of London
London, United Kingdom

Ananda Datta
Department of Pulmonary Medicine
    and Critical Care
All India Institute of Medical
    Sciences
Bhubaneswar, India

Mantu Jain
Department of Orthopaedics
All India Institute of Medical Sciences
Bhubaneswar, India

Menka Jha
Department of Neurology
All India Institute of Medical Sciences
Bhubaneswar, India

Pankaj Kumar
Department of Surgery
All India Institute of Medical Sciences
Bhubaneswar, India

Rudra Pratap Mahapatra
Department of Cardiothoracic and
    Vascular Surgery
All India Institute of Medical Sciences
Bhubaneswar, India

Baijayantimala Mishra
Department of Microbiology
All India Institute of Medical Sciences
Bhubaneswar, India

Narayan Prasad Mishra
Department of Orthopaedics
All India Institute of Medical
    Sciences
Bhubaneswar, India

Srujana Mohanty
Department of Microbiology
All India Institute of Medical
    Sciences
Bhubaneswar, India

Prasanta R Mohapatra
Department of Pulmonary Medicine
    and Critical Care
All India Institute of Medical Sciences
Bhubaneswar, India

Suprava Naik
Department of Radiodiagnosis
All India Institute of Medical Sciences
Bhubaneswar, India

Hemanta K Nayak
Department of Gastroenterology
All India Institute of Medical Sciences
Bhubaneswar, India

Manas K Panigrahi
Department of Gastroenterology
All India Institute of Medical Sciences
Bhubaneswar, India

Ranjan Kumar Patel
Department of Radiodiagnosis
All India Institute of Medical Sciences
Bhubaneswar, India

Abhijeet Rai
Department of Gastroenterology
All India Institute of Medical Sciences
Bhubaneswar, India

Arpita Nibedita Rout
Department of Dermatology
All India Institute of Medical Sciences
Bhubaneswar, India

Prakash K Sasmal
Department of Surgery
All India Institute of Medical Sciences
Bhubaneswar, India

Chandra Sekhar Sirka
Department of Dermatology
All India Institute of Medical Sciences
Bhubaneswar, India

Sujit Kumar Tripathy
Department of Orthopaedics
All India Institute of Medical
    Sciences
Bhubaneswar, India

Melioidosis in Global Perspective and Challenges for Surveillance

1

David AB Dance

Centre for Tropical Medicine & Global Health, University of Oxford, Oxford, United Kingdom

London School of Hygiene and Tropical Medicine, University of London, London, United Kingdom

Contents

INTRODUCTION

For many decades, melioidosis was regarded as a rare disease of little significance, confined to certain remote parts of the tropics. Over the past 40 years, it has emerged as an infection with important implications for global public health, both as an understanding

DOI: 10.1201/9781003324010-1

of its true distribution and burden has grown and as its potential as a biothreat agent has been explored. In this chapter, I will briefly review the 'known knowns' and the 'known unknowns' as far as melioidosis is concerned, explore some of the obstacles to unravelling the latter, and, finally, consider whether melioidosis, which is so neglected that it is not even on the World Health Organization's (WHO) list of neglected tropical diseases (NTDs), should be formally recognized as such.

WORLDWIDE DISTRIBUTION AND DISSEMINATION

Back in 1991, I reviewed what was then known about the worldwide distribution of melioidosis from literature.[1] At this time, it was clear that the disease was endemic throughout Southeast Asia and in northern Australia, but there were tantalizing glimpses of endemicity elsewhere throughout the tropics. Over the ensuing 30 years, endemicity in many of these places has been confirmed by the detection of human or animal infections and the presence of *Burkholderia pseudomallei* in the environment. The situation was reviewed again in 2016, when 45 countries were identified as endemic and another 34 were highlighted as potentially endemic because of a favourable climate and environment for *B. pseudomallei*.[2] Since that paper was published, evidence supporting endemicity has been found in several of these 34 countries, including Nepal,[3–6] Benin,[7] Cameroon,[8] Democratic Republic of Congo,[9] Eritrea,[10] Ghana,[11,12] Mali,[13] Nicaragua,[14] Saint Kitts and Nevis,[15] Trinidad and Tobago,[16] the Federated States of Micronesia,[17] and, most recently, the southern United States (US).[18,19]

Whenever melioidosis is identified in a new location, the question inevitably arises as to whether it has long been present but unrecognized or whether it has been recently introduced, for example, by international travel of infected humans or animals or transported by contaminated products or objects. All of these are theoretically possible, but the extent to which they can lead to the establishment of new endemic foci is unknown. Infection in returning travellers is well described and extensively reviewed.[20–22] Infections in animals or fish imported from endemic areas into non-endemic areas have also been frequently reported and have sometimes given rise to considerable public health concerns and occasional human infections.[23,24] A striking recent example of melioidosis resulting from the importation of a contaminated product is the cluster of four cases, two of whom died, across the US in 2021, which was eventually traced back to a contaminated aromatherapy spray manufactured in India.[25]

The advent of modern genomic techniques has provided fascinating insights into the global dissemination and timelines of *B. pseudomallei* transmission. The degree of diversity amongst clinical and environmental isolates can reveal the length of time the organism has been present in a newly recognized environment.[17] It appears that the species originated in Australia,[26] from where it has spread multiple times into Southeast Asia and thence onto Africa and the Americas, the latter around the time of the slave trade.[27,28] However, this is not one-way traffic: a particular sequence type of *B. pseudomallei*,

ST562, appears to have been introduced from southern China into the Darwin region of northern Australia sometime around 1988, since when it has caused an increasing proportion of human and animal melioidosis in the Darwin area.[29] No doubt, the widespread application of whole-genome sequencing to isolates from around the world will shed further light on the precise dynamics of *B. pseudomallei* spread in the future.

DISEASE BURDEN

The 2016 modelling paper by Limmathurotsakul et al. has become one of the most widely cited papers in the field, as it contains the best estimate we have of the total global melioidosis burden: 165,000 human cases (95% credible interval 68,000–412,000) and 89,000 (36,000–227,000) deaths per year worldwide.[2] Notably, some 44% of these cases were predicted to occur in South Asia, particularly India. When further analysed to estimate the burden in terms of disability-adjusted life years (DALYs), this equated to 4.6 million DALYs (uncertainty interval 3.2–6.6) or 84.3 per 100,000 people (57.5–120.0), the majority of which was accounted for by the high mortality rate.[30]

Nonetheless, like any model, this study was based on a series of assumptions, particularly about the features of an environment that make it suitable for the survival of *B. pseudomallei* in soil and water, which may or may not prove to be correct. Our understanding of the complex interactions between the bacterium and the physical, chemical, and biological characteristics of its various ecological niches is rudimentary. So, it would not be surprising if some of the projections proved to be wrong. This is at least partly due to the difficulty of detecting *B. pseudomallei* reliably in environmental samples and the need to consider the extreme structural complexity and micro-niches within soil.[31] Assumptions about the proportion of the exposed population who become infected and die may also be wrong. Thus, the model needs to be continually refined as more data become available.

In fact, the numbers of cases that have been reported, either through national surveillance systems or in the literature, fall well short of the number of cases predicted by the modelling, as a series of national and regional reviews published in 2019 clearly demonstrate.[32] This is particularly marked for India, where less than 1,000 cases were identified from the literature and local records, as opposed to more than 50,000 cases annually nationwide predicted by the model, a dramatic discrepancy. In countries with well-resourced healthcare systems and mandatory surveillance, such as Singapore and Australia, however, the number of cases reported comes far closer to the numbers predicted by the modelling.

Whether the numbers from the model are anywhere near the truth remains to be determined. The extent to which melioidosis can pass below the radar is amply illustrated by the example of the Lao People's Democratic Republic (Laos). This country lies across the Mekong River from northeast Thailand, where melioidosis has been known to be highly endemic for many years.[33] When a research collaboration was established in 1999 between the University of Oxford and Mahosot Hospital in the capital, Vientiane, melioidosis had never previously been diagnosed in Laos. Within two years, cases had begun to be recognized,[34] and by 2017, 1539 cases had been microbiologically confirmed.[35] It is highly unlikely that the disease had not existed within Laos before 1999, and whilst, of course, it is possible that factors such as climate change and, an increased prevalence and longer survival of patients with predisposing conditions such as diabetes mellitus might have led to a genuine increase in melioidosis incidence, it is far more likely that the disease was simply being missed. Since most of these 1539 cases were diagnosed in Vientiane, the only city that at that time had a comprehensive diagnostic microbiology service, it is also likely that many cases of melioidosis are still being missed elsewhere within Laos.

BARRIERS TO SURVEILLANCE

There are multiple barriers to gaining accurate data on the number of cases of melioidosis in each country, as illustrated in Figure 1.1.

The first barrier is access to healthcare. Trained healthcare workers are unevenly distributed, and diagnostic laboratories even more so, and they are especially scarce in the remote rural areas where melioidosis patients are likely to live. Even if laboratories do exist, in countries where patients have to pay for diagnostic tests, poor subsistence rice farmers are unlikely to be able to afford to pay for these.

Secondly, awareness of melioidosis is poor in many countries amongst both clinicians and laboratory staff (and even more so amongst the general public).[36] Even if physicians know of the disease, the clinical manifestations of melioidosis are many and varied, giving rise to the nickname 'the great mimicker (or imitator)',[37] so diagnosis on

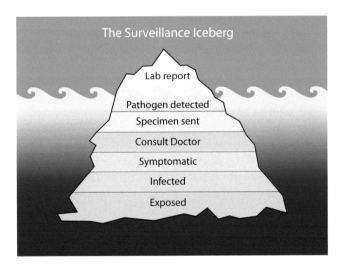

FIGURE 1.1 The surveillance iceberg, showing that the cases of an infection reported to national surveillance systems or in the literature may represent only a small proportion of the total number of cases occurring. (Reproduced with permission from *Melioidosis: A Century of Observation and Research*, Edited by N. Ketheesan. © 2012 Elsevier B.V.)

clinical grounds alone is unreliable, meaning that laboratory confirmation is necessary for accurate diagnosis and surveillance. However, since laboratory staff are often not trained in the identification of environmental organisms such as *B. pseudomallei*, the literature is littered with instances in which the diagnosis has been missed or delayed, often with fatal results, even when appropriate samples had been taken and the organism had been isolated but either dismissed or misidentified.[38–41]

Finally, even if the patient has managed to see a doctor who has sent appropriate samples and the laboratory has isolated and correctly identified the organism, it may or may not be captured by local surveillance systems. Even in countries where mandatory laboratory-based surveillance systems exist, official data regarding melioidosis can be grossly misleading. For example, it has been known since the mid-1980s that melioidosis is highly endemic in Thailand, especially in the northeast part of the country.[33] Nonetheless, when Hantrakun and colleagues reviewed 7126 laboratory-confirmed cases between 2012 and 2015, they found major discrepancies between the laboratory data and what was being reported through the National Notifiable Diseases Surveillance System (NNDSS), particularly over-reporting of cases based on serology, which is notoriously inaccurate, and dramatic under-reporting of deaths.[42] Even in a country like the United Kingdom (UK), where melioidosis is not endemic and the number of cases seen is small, and where notification of the isolation of *B. pseudomallei* by laboratories became mandatory under the Health Protection (Notification) Regulations 2010, O'Connor et al. found that only 19 of 46 (41.3%) patients with culture-confirmed melioidosis diagnosed in the UK between January 2010 and July 2019 had been notified.[43]

BIOTHREAT POTENTIAL

B. pseudomallei is one of the bacteria that has been considered as an agent that might be used as a weapon, either by terrorists or by state actors. It was classified as a 'Category B critical biological agent for public health preparedness' by Rotz et al. in 2002,[44] and more recently as a 'Tier 1 Select Agent' by the US Department of Health and Human Services and Department of Agriculture (https://www.selectagents.gov/sat/list.htm). The reasons for this are several-fold. First, *Burkholderia mallei*, the causative agent of glanders, which is effectively a clone of *B. pseudomallei* that has become adapted as a pathogen of equines in association with the loss of large sections of its genome,[45] was used as a weapon against horses by German agents during World War I.[46] Secondly, *B. pseudomallei* is known to be infectious by inhalation, and in animal models the infectious dose can be extremely low. Thirdly, it is intrinsically resistant to antibiotics and difficult to treat. Additionally, as an environmental saprophyte that is widespread in tropical environments, it would be relatively easy to obtain. On the other hand, there appears to have been little research done into its weaponization, at least as far as is known from information in the public domain, although it was undoubtedly an agent of interest to Biopreparat, the Soviet biological weapons programme.[47] It would certainly not be as easy to aerosolize as a spore-forming organism like *Bacillus anthracis* and, as an opportunistic pathogen with a predilection for people with underlying conditions such as diabetes mellitus, its impact on whole populations is difficult to predict. This topic has been extensively reviewed.[46]

Nonetheless, whether or not *B. pseudomallei* is likely ever to be used as a weapon, the attention paid to the organism undoubtedly increased after its classification as a Select Agent, as did the funding devoted to melioidosis research, so this has not been without its benefits to melioidosis as a real-world public health problem.

MELIOIDOSIS AS A NEGLECTED TROPICAL DISEASE

Suppose the predictions from the model of Limmathurotsakul et al. are anywhere near accurate. In that case, the annual global mortality from melioidosis is comparable to that of measles and higher than some infections that are far better known, such as leptospirosis and dengue.[2] The overall disease burden would be considerably higher than that of many diseases that are formally classified as NTDs by the WHO and falls primarily on the rural poor working in agriculture.[30] It is certainly greatly under-diagnosed and, therefore, inappropriately treated, but if detected early and treated correctly, mortality can be reduced from around 50% to less than 10%.[48] This recently led several of us to call for the WHO to recognize melioidosis as an 'official' NTD in the hope that this would further raise the profile of the infection and result in it being given higher priority by local and global health agencies.[49]

CONCLUSIONS

Whatever the true burden and distribution of melioidosis eventually proves to be, there is no doubt that it is currently grossly under-recognized and under-reported. It fulfils the criteria for an NTD, and it is long overdue that it should be formally recognized as such. Only better surveillance, improved access to diagnostics, better education of clinicians and laboratory staff in its recognition and management, and the implementation of effective preventive measures will help to reduce the unnecessary suffering and death toll from this silent killer.

REFERENCES

1. Dance DAB. Melioidosis: The Tip of the Iceberg? Clin Microbiol Rev 1991; 4(1): 52–60.
2. Limmathurotsakul D, et al. Predicted Global Distribution of *Burkholderia pseudomallei* and Burden of Melioidosis. Nat Microbiol 2016; 1: 15008.
3. Parajuli S, et al. Bilateral Non Granulomatous Anterior Uveitis from Melioidosis Case Report. Acta Sci Ophthalmol 2020; 3(8): 3–5.

4. Kuijpers SC, et al. Primary Cutaneous Melioidosis Acquired in Nepal – Case Report and Literature Review. Travel Med Infect Dis 2021; 42: 102080.

5. Bhandari PB, et al. A Fatal Case of Cerebral Melioidosis. Med J Shree Birendra Hosp 2019; 18(2): 64–68.

6. Abu Khattab M, et al. Melioidosis an Imported Infection in Qatar: Case Series and Literature Review. Adv Infect Dis 2022; 12(2): 175–92.

7. Ombelet S, et al. Blood Culture Surveillance in a Secondary Care Hospital in Benin: Epidemiology of Bloodstream Infection Pathogens and Antimicrobial Resistance. BMC Infect Dis 2022; 22: 119. https://doi.org/10.1186/s12879-022-07077-z.

8. Bousquet A, et al. Accidental Exposure to *Burkholderia pseudomallei*: Awareness Is Also Needed for Urine Specimens. Clin Microbiol Infect 2020; 26(2): 265–66.

9. Shongo MY-P, et al. Melioidosis and Sickle Cell Disease: Description of a Rare Association. Theory Clin Pract Pediatr 2020; 3(1): 57–62.

10. Almog Y, et al. A *Burkholderia pseudomallei* Infection Imported from Eritrea to Israel. Am J Trop Med Hyg 2016; 95(5): 997–98.

11. Oduro G, et al. On the Environmental Presence of *Burkholderia pseudomallei* in South-Central Ghana. Appl Environ Microbiol 2022; 88(12): e0060022.

12. Mabayoje DA, et al. Melioidosis Manifesting as Chronic Femoral Osteomyelitis in Patient from Ghana. Emerg Infect Dis 2022; 28(1): 201–04.

13. Dicko AA, et al. Mélioïdose Cutanée: A Propos d'un Cas Au Mali. Revue Malienne d'Infectiologie et de Microbiologie 2022; 17(1): 97–99.

14. Pasupneti T, et al. Disseminated Melioidosis in a Patient from Nicaragua. IDCases 2021; 26: e01318.

15. Canales R, et al. Melioidosis in a Bottlenose Dolphin (Tursiops Truncatus) After a Hurricane in the Caribbean Islands. J Zoo Wildl Med 2020; 51(2): 443–47.

16. Hogan C, et al. Melioidosis in Trinidad and Tobago. Emerg Infect Dis 2015; 21(5): 902–04.

17. Nolen LD, et al. Differentiating New from Newly Detected: Melioidosis in Yap, Federated States of Micronesia. Am J Trop Med Hyg 2019; 101(2): 323–27. https://doi.org/10.4269/ajtmh.19-0253.

18. CDC Health Alert Network. Melioidosis Locally Endemic in Areas of the Mississippi Gulf Coast after *Burkholderia pseudomallei* Isolated in Soil and Water and Linked to Two Cases – Mississippi, 2020 and 2022. https://www.google.com/url?sa=t&rct=j&q=&esrc=s&source=web&cd=&ved=2ahUKEwjgoID27a_5AhXxRkEAHY3sC2gQFnoECBAQAQ&url=https%3A%2F%2Fwww.emergency.cdc.gov%2Fhan%2F2022%2Fpdf%2FCDC_HAN_470.pdf&usg=AOvVaw0EHqQWY5IUIWfTpi5PZka_(accessed 05/08/22).

19. Cossaboom CM, et al. Melioidosis in a Resident of Texas with No Recent Travel History, United States. Emerg Infect Dis 2020; 26(6): 1295–99.

20. Dan M. Melioidosis in Travelers: Review of the Literature. J Travel Med 2015; 22(6): 410–14.

21. Birnie E, et al. Melioidosis in Travelers: An Analysis of Dutch Melioidosis Registry Data 1985-2018. Travel Med Infect Dis 2019: 101461. https://doi.org/10.1016/j.tmaid.2019.07.017.

22. Saidani N, et al. Melioidosis as a Travel-Associated Infection: Case Report and Review of the Literature. Travel Med Infect Dis 2015; 13(5): 367–81.

23. Ryan CW, et al. Public Health Response to an Imported Case of Canine Melioidosis. Zoonoses Public Health 2018; 65(4): 420–24.

24. Dawson P, et al. Human Melioidosis Caused by Novel Transmission of *Burkholderia pseudomallei* from Freshwater Home Aquarium, United States(1). Emerg Infect Dis 2021; 27(12): 3030–35.

25. Gee JE, et al. Multistate Outbreak of Melioidosis Associated with Imported Aromatherapy Spray. N Engl J Med 2022; 386(9): 861–68.

26. Pearson T, et al. Phylogeographic Reconstruction of a Bacterial Species with High Levels of Lateral Gene Transfer. BMC Biology 2009; 7: 78.

27. Sarovich DS, et al. Phylogenomic Analysis Reveals an Asian Origin for African *Burkholderia pseudomallei* and Further Supports Melioidosis Endemicity in Africa. mSphere 2016; 1(2) e00089-15. https://doi.org/10.1128/mSphere.00089-15.

28. Chewapreecha C, et al. Global and Regional Dissemination and Evolution of *Burkholderia pseudomallei*. Nat Microbiol 2017; 2: 162–63.

29. Meumann EM, et al. Emergence of *Burkholderia pseudomallei* Sequence Type 562, Northern Australia. Emerg Infect Dis 2021; 27(4): 1057–67.

30. Birnie E, et al. Global Burden of Melioidosis in 2015: A Systematic Review and Data Synthesis. Lancet Infect Dis 2019; 19(8): 892–902.

31. Manivanh L, et al. *Burkholderia pseudomallei* in a Lowland Rice Paddy: Seasonal Changes and Influence of Soil Depth and Physico-Chemical Properties. Sci Rep 2017; 7(1): 3031.

32. Direk Limmathurotsakul and David AB Dance. Global burden and challenges of melioidosis. Basel: MDPI; 2019.

33. Suputtamongkol Y, et al. The Epidemiology of Melioidosis in Ubon Ratchatani, Northeast Thailand. Int J Epidemiol 1994; 23(5): 1082–90.

34. Phetsouvanh R, et al. Melioidosis and Pandora's Box in the Lao People's Democratic Republic. Clin Infect Dis 2001; 32(4): 653–54.

35. Dance DAB, et al. Melioidosis in the Lao People's Democratic Republic. Trop Med Infect Dis 2018; 3(1): 21. https://doi.org/10.3390/tropicalmed3010021.

36. Chansrichavala P, et al. Public Awareness of Melioidosis in Thailand and Potential Use of Video Clips as Educational Tools. PLoS One [Electronic Resource] 2015; 10(3): e0121311.

37. Yee KC, et al. Melioidosis, the Great Mimicker: A Report of 10 Cases from Malaysia. Am J Trop Med Hyg 1988; 91(5): 249–54.

38. Muthumbi EM, et al. Population-Based Estimate of Melioidosis. Kenya Emerg Infect Dis 2019; 25(5): 984–87.

39. Wu B, et al. Misidentification of *Burkholderia pseudomallei*, China. Emerg Infect Dis 2021; 27(3): 964–66.

40. Nguyen HB, et al. Case of Misdiagnosed Melioidosis from Hue City, Vietnam. Iran J Microbiol 2022; 14(3): 430–33.

41. Greer RC, et al. Misidentification of *Burkholderia pseudomallei* as *Acinetobacter* species in Northern Thailand. Trans R Soc Trop Med Hyg 2019; 113(1): 48–51.

42. Hantrakun V, et al. Clinical Epidemiology of 7126 Melioidosis Patients in Thailand and the Implications for a National Notifiable Diseases Surveillance System. Open Forum Infect Dis 2019; 6(12): ofz498.

43. O'Connor C, et al. Imported Melioidosis in the United Kingdom: Increasing Incidence but Continued Under-Reporting. Clin Infect Pract 2020: 100051.

44. Rotz LD, et al. Public Health Assessment of Potential Biological Terrorism Agents. Emerg Infect Dis 2002; 8(2): 225–30.

45. Nierman WC, et al. Structural Flexibility in the *Burkholderia mallei* Genome. Proc Natl Acad Sci USA 2004; 101(39): 14246–51.

46. Dance DAB. Melioidosis and glanders as possible biological weapons. In: Fong I, Alibek K, eds. Bioterrorism and infectious agents: a new dilemma for the 21st century. New York: Springer; 2005: 99–145.

47. Alibek K. Biohazard: the chilling true story of the largest covert biological weapons program in the world, told from the inside by the man who ran it: first edition. New York: Random House; 1999.

48. Currie BJ, et al. The Darwin Prospective Melioidosis Study: A 30-Year Prospective, Observational Investigation. Lancet Infect Dis 2021; 21(12): 1737–46.

49. Savelkoel J, et al. A Call to Action: Time to Recognise Melioidosis as a Neglected Tropical Disease. Lancet Infect Dis 2022; 22(6): e176–82.

Epidemiology of Melioidosis

2

Baijayantimala Mishra

Department of Microbiology, All India Institute of Medical Sciences, Bhubaneswar, India

Contents

The soil and water in tropical countries act as the natural reservoir of *Burkholderia pseudomallei*. Humans acquire the infection through inoculation, ingestion, and inhalation. Most cases are reported during the monsoon months, possibly acquired from contaminated soil through percutaneous inoculation. Heavy rainfall with high winds has been associated with severe melioidosis. Though the infection can occur in all age groups and both genders, most cases are seen in adult males 45–60 years of age. Diabetes mellitus, chronic kidney impairment, other chronic organ dysfunctions, and iron overloading conditions like thalassemia are important risk factors. Increased temperature, changes in environmental precipitation patterns in a tropical country, and increased extreme weather events are expected to change melioidosis epidemiology.

An estimated 3 billion people live in the area likely to harbour *B. pseudomallei*. Due to gross under-reporting or non-reporting of cases, the exact global burden of melioidosis is not known.

DOI: 10.1201/9781003324010-2

In a modelling study, the estimated global burden of human melioidosis has been predicted as 165,000 cases against the annual reported cases of 1300 per year since 2010, with a mortality rate of 54%, amounting to 89,000 annual deaths worldwide.[1]

Melioidosis is prevalent in Southeast Asian countries and northern Australia. It is endemic in 45 countries, where it is still grossly under-reported and expected to be potentially endemic in additional 34 countries, which are yet to report indigenous cases.[1]

Australia: Melioidosis is endemic in the northern regions of Australia, north of 20°S latitude, and some focal parts of southern temperate regions latitude 30°S. The annual incidence ranges from 5.4 to 41.7 per 100,000, with an average of 19.6 cases.[2]

During the wet monsoon season of 2009–2010, with above-average rainfall, Australia recorded 50.2 cases/100,000 population and 102.4 cases/100,000 population among the Top-end indigenous population, the highest ever documented annual incidence in the world.[3]

The average annual incidence in the Torres Straight Islands, Cape York, and Cairns is 33.1, 12.1, and 1.7/100,000, respectively.[4] Several melioidosis cases in humans and animals have been documented in Australia relating to unchlorinated water contaminated with *B. pseudomallei.*

Southeast Asia: Thailand – Geographically, *B. pseudomallei* is likely to be present throughout Thailand, and the disease is expected to be endemic throughout the country. The annual incidence of human melioidosis cases has been estimated in a modelling study as 7572, with a mortality rate of 37%, amounting to 2838 deaths.[1] Melioidosis is endemic predominantly in the northeast part of the country, which is the largest region of Thailand, with 20 provinces.

The endemicity in southern Thailand is gradually becoming recognized. Several cases were reported in tsunami survivors in 2004 in Phang Nga on the west coast. During 2002–2011, 134 culture-proven cases were reported from Hat Yai, where 37% of cases were bacteraemic, and fatality was 7%. In 2012, an outbreak of 11 cases consisting of 8 Thais and 3 foreign tourists was reported in Koh Pha Ngan, an island on the east coast of southern Thailand.[5–7]

Historically, eastern, western, and central Thailand are not considered to be endemic for melioidosis.[8] However, the evidence regarding the existence of the causative bacterium and endemicity has gradually accumulated. In population-based surveillance during 2006–2008 in Sa Kaeo province in East Thailand, the estimated average incidence of bacteraemia melioidosis was 4.9 cases per 100,000 population, with a population mortality rate of 1.9 per 100,000.[9]

Vietnam recorded its first human case in 1927, and after that, several hundred human cases were reported in French and American soldiers during their deployment in Vietnam. Most of these cases have been diagnosed in modern hospitals in Vietnam or the United States.[10] The concept of latent melioidosis and reactivation came after a few cases were reported in US soldiers years after their return from Vietnam, which led to the name of the 'Vietnamese time bomb' for melioidosis. The report of melioidosis among the indigenous Vietnamese is much less possible due to a lack of microbiological diagnostic facilities. In 2014, a research network on melioidosis and *B. pseudomallei* was started, and after this, 70 cases were detected within seven months with a detection rate of 3.4%–10.2% among the positive blood cultures.[10] *B. pseudomallei* is present all over Vietnam, as evident by the isolates from 80% of soil samples, a high number of clinical cases, and seroprevalence of up to 31.8%.[11]

Laos: Melioidosis is highly endemic in Laos, though still grossly under-reported. In 1999, a research collaboration was established, and the Lao-Oxford-Mahosot Hospital Wellcome Trust Research Unit (LOWMRU) was created to support the diagnosis of melioidosis. Since then, the number of reported cases has been increasing every year. With further support from Centre d'Infectiologie Christophe Mérieux du Laos and European Union, the diagnostic microbiology in Laos is becoming more developed and capable of diagnosing melioidosis. In a review published in 2018, more than 1300 cases were reported from various parts of Laos between 1999 and 2017. Recently, more than 100 cases have been reported every year only from Mahosot Hospital. The causative bacterium *B. pseudomallei* has been found to be widespread in soil and water.[12]

Myanmar: Though the disease melioidosis was first recognized in Rangoon, Myanmar (previously Burma), in 1911 by the British pathologist Whitmore, the disease was hardly reported thereafter for more than 50 years. Whitmore had reported 38 post-mortem cases of glander-like disease, and Krishnaswami in 1917 reported that he had seen 200 cases in six years. However, due to political turmoil, the diagnostic and research development was affected for several decades, and the cases have only been sporadically reported in the country. In a 2018 review, a total of 298 cases were reported since 1913, whereas 258 cases were before 1948, and the majority (>90%) of cases belonged to Yangon (formerly Rangoon). The modelling study by Limmathurotsakul et al. has predicted an annual number of 6000 cases and 3000 deaths.[1]

However, a report of 3865 blood cultures from 2005 to 2013 in a major hospital in Yangon found that *B. pseudomallei* was not isolated, which the authors attributed to a sub-optimal diagnostic technique.

Malaysia and **Singapore** are both endemic to melioidosis and report many melioidosis cases. The number of annual cases in Malaysia is suggested in the range of 1.6–16.4 per 100,000 population, with an estimated annual death of 2000 cases. The causative bacterium has been isolated in soil and water from various parts of Malaysia. The human cases have been reported mostly from the states where agriculture is the major economic activity.[13] On the contrary, the overall incidence in Singapore is 1.1 per 100,000 population with a decreasing trend in the yearly incidence rate of 10%. In a 12-year study in Singapore, the incidence was higher among the Malay and Indian populations than in the local population. The seroprevalence also shows a significantly higher rate among the non-Singapore workers from neighbouring Malaysia, Thailand, and India than the local workers. The isolation rate from soil and water is also lower in Singapore than in the other endemic Southeast Asian countries.[14]

Africa and Americas: Occasional indigenous cases have been reported from Africa and the Americas. A significant part of Africa is endemic to melioidosis but is mostly under-reported or never reported. It is suggested that *B. pseudomallei* is widely distributed across the countries. The predicted incidence in Nigeria alone is 13,400 per year. Recently, Ghana has reported a case of chronic osteomyelitis and isolation of *B. pseudomallei* from the soil in rice farms. With the WHO's effort to create awareness and laboratory support, it is expected to get more reported cases in times to come.

Isolates from different regions of South America show high genomic diversity. Recently, Brazil has reported a high proportion of paediatric melioidosis with severe disease. The southern United States comes under the predicted endemic area for melioidosis, and the causative bacterium *B. pseudomallei* has recently been reported from the US Virgin Islands. In 2022, a multi-state outbreak of melioidosis cases in the United States was traced to a contaminated aroma therapy spray imported from India.

South Asia: The predicted contribution of cases from South Asian countries where melioidosis is not considered endemic is 44% of the global burden, which is higher in contrast to 40% in East Asia and the Pacific region, where melioidosis is known to be prevalent. The predicted rate of cases in India, Indonesia, and Bangladesh are ~52,500, ~20,000, and ~16,900 cases per year, respectively. The contribution of South Asia, particularly the Indian sub-continent, was estimated to be higher, as a large population resides in this region, which is contaminated with *B. pseudomallei*. Increasing cases are being reported from various parts of India. Increasing awareness among medical microbiologists and clinicians has increased the number of reported cases, particularly during the last decade. The majority of the reported cases are from the south and eastern coastal states like Tamil Nadu, Kerala, Karnataka, and Odisha. However, in recent years, several cases have been reported almost from all parts of the country except a few northern states.[15,16] Sri Lanka and Bangladesh are considered to be endemic; however, melioidosis still remains highly under-detected in these countries.

THE AGENT

B. pseudomallei is a small Gram-negative environmental bacteria present in the soil and water in the endemic regions. The organism closely resembles the members of the genus *Pseudomonas*; it was previously called *Pseudomonas pseudomallei*.

Molecular Epidemiology

This high heterogenicity of the genome across *B. pseudomallei* strains is likely responsible for varied disease manifestations and disease courses of melioidosis.

Phylogenetic analysis demonstrates that isolates of Australasia and Asia are distinct. The genetic diversity of Australasia is more than that of Asian isolates. This indicates Australia was an early reservoir for the current global *B. pseudomallei* population.[17]

Among the Asian isolates, the Mekong subregion, the border region of the Mekong River, is considered a hot spot for *B. pseudomallei* evolution compared to isolates from Malaysia and Singapore.[17] Isolates from Africa and Central and South America appear to have a common origin in Africa. The introduction of *B. pseudomallei* from Africa to South America coincides with the peak of the slave trade during the 17th and 19th centuries.[17]

ENVIRONMENT AND MELIOIDOSIS

B. pseudomallei is an environmental bacteria present in the soil, water, and air. The presence of bacteria depends on the soil type, moisture content of the soil, water drainage capacity, temperature, pH, and salinity, etc. Waterlogged soils, arthrosol (heavily modified by human activity), and acrisol soil (clay-rich) types having a moisture content more than 40% are positively associated with the persistence of the bacteria for more than two years. However, northeast Thailand, which is endemic to melioidosis, contains mostly sandy soil and has also been shown to support the survival of the bacteria. This is possibly due to the free flow of the water up and down through the sandy soil. Hence, it is not only the type of soil but also the moisture content, temperature, salinity, pH, nitrogen content, etc., that affect the overall persistence of *B. pseudomallei* in the soil. Moreover, the bacteria exist more than 30 cm deep in the soil and during the rainy season (Table 2.1) ploughing the bacteria-infested land during plantation helps the bacteria come in contact with humans, leading to more cases in the wet months. Across endemic countries, more than 70% of melioidosis cases are reported during the rainy season. Monsoon increases the *B. pseudomallei* load on the soil surface and also its survival, leading to an increased chance of percutaneous inoculation while working in muddy soil. Heavy rainfall has been shown to be an independent predictor of severe melioidosis when it occurs a few weeks prior to hospital presentation. A possibility of acquiring infection through the inhalation route has been hypothesized in this context as intense rainfall is usually associated with heavy wind, leading to aerosolization of bacteria from surface soil. Detection of non-cultivable *B. pseudomallei* DNA from dry superficial soils indicates the possibility of the existence of the bacteria in a viable but non-cultivable state.

Cloud cover is considered another important determinant of the rise in several cases. A dense layer of clouds indicates the wet season, increases moisture, and protects the bacteria from ultraviolet light, thereby facilitating the survival of *B. pseudomallei*.

The effect of La Niña leading to increased sea-surface temperature, high evaporation and humidity, and early and strong monsoon has been noted more than once in North Australia. Clusters of cases have been reported after extreme weather events like cyclones and typhoons.[18,19]

TABLE 2.1   Environmental predictor of melioidosis

Humidity
Rainfall
Wind speed
Exposure to agriculture and farming are prominent
Anthrosol (heavily modified with organic waste) and acrisol (clay-rich associated with humid, tropical climates) soil encountered in irrigated agriculture
Residual crop burning results in depletion of soil nutrients
Exposure to soil

The occurrence of melioidosis cases, however, depends on the complex interaction between weather, soil type, flora, fauna, and human population.

MELIOIDOSIS AND ANIMALS

Melioidosis has been documented in more than 50 species of terrestrial and aquatic animals, including birds and fish. The clinical manifestations varied from asymptomatic to fatal septicaemia. The disease is more susceptible in sheep, alpacas, and camels, whereas goats may present variedly. Outbreaks have been reported in livestock animals such as pigs, cattle, goats, and captive animals. In general, animals in endemic countries are considered relatively resistant to infection compared to the exotic captive animals in the non-endemic locality. Transmission from an infected animal to a human and vice versa is not well established. *B. pseudomallei* has been isolated in faecal samples of chicken and wallabies and beaks of healthy native birds, which may play a role in the geographical dissemination of the bacteria.[20]

MODES OF TRANSMISSION

Percutaneous inoculation, ingestion, and inhalation are the three major routes of transmission. Inoculation through contaminated soil is considered the most common mode of transmission as the disease is more common in rural populations working in soil or mostly in waterlogged agriculture fields, and the maximum number of cases are reported during the monsoon months as the condition becomes more favourable for the bacteria, which comes to the surface due to ploughing (Figure 2.1).

The acquisition of infection through ingestion of contaminated water was initially thought to be common in grazing animals and not an important transmission route for humans. However, a few outbreaks reported from the rural areas of Thailand and the northern territory of Australia were established due to ingestion of contaminated unchlorinated water supply based on the genetic relatedness between the strain found in water and the infected cases.[21–23] Acute suppurative parotitis in Thai children has been attributed to direct ingestion of the bacteria,[24] and an acute parotitis in children was found using drinking water from the same well.[25] Ingestion of breast milk from a mother with melioidosis also has been reported as a possible mode of transmission.[26] Nosocomial transmission through contaminated wound irrigation fluid, hand-washing, and antiseptics has also been documented.[27,28]

Inhalation of aerosolized dry dust containing suspended *B. pseudomallei* particles was thought to be a mode of transmission of *B. pseudomallei* when many American helicopter crew members were infected after the Vietnam War. This and the disease's long incubation period led to the epithet 'Vietnamese time bomb.' Epidemiological evidence

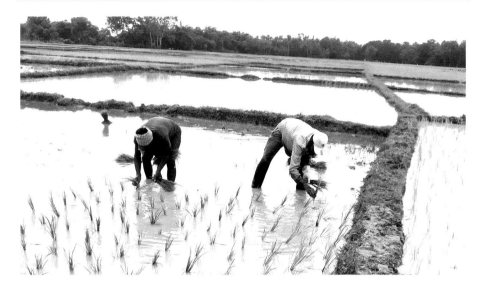

FIGURE 2.1 Exposure to mud close to a water surface or muddy areas in the rice fields during plantation.

from North Australia has shown more pneumonic melioidosis and severe disease during the rainy season when heavy rain is accompanied by strong winds leading to the possibility of inhalation as a route of acquisition.[2]

However, pulmonary melioidosis can occur even when the bacteria are acquired through inoculation. There is no direct evidence of human-to-human transmission via the respiratory route of transmission or transmission to close contacts of a patient with pulmonary melioidosis.

Though inoculation, ingestion, and inhalation are the three accepted modes of transmission, the exact event of time, place, and route of infection is usually difficult to establish in individual cases.

HOST FACTORS

Melioidosis affects all ages and both sexes. However, most cases occur between the age of 40 and 60, with a male preponderance of about 80% or more. Several risk factors are associated with melioidosis, like diabetes mellitus, chronic renal failure, excess alcohol consumption, chronic lung disease, chronic liver disease, thalassemia, and immunosuppression (Table 2.2). Of all the risk factors, diabetes mellitus is the most common risk factor, which is found in more than 50% of melioidosis cases, and persons with diabetes mellitus are 12 times more at risk of developing the disease.

TABLE 2.2 Risk factors for melioidosis

Diabetes
Chronic renal impairment
Heavy alcohol intake
Chronic lung disease
Chronic liver disease
Chronic heart disease
Thalassemia
Immunosuppression
Prolonged steroid intake

CONCLUSION

Melioidosis is predicted to be endemic in most tropical countries. The current reported cases are highly under-detected due to a lack of awareness among microbiologists and clinicians. With increasing efforts to create awareness, more cases are being reported. More genomic analysis reveals the causative bacteria's origin, spread, and evolution. However, continuous efforts towards this would bring out the real epidemiological scenario, which is essential to take necessary preventive measures to save lives of this fatal disease.

REFERENCES

1. Limmathurotsakul D, et al. Predicted Global Distribution of *Burkholderia pseudomallei* and Burden of Melioidosis. Nat Microbiol 2016; 1(1): 15008.
2. Cheng AC, et al. Melioidosis: Epidemiology, Pathophysiology, and Management. Clin Microbiol Rev 2005; 18(2): 383–416.
3. Parameswaran U, et al. Melioidosis at Royal Darwin Hospital in the Big 2009-2010 Wet Season: Comparison with the Preceding 20 Years. Med J Aust 2012; 196(5): 345–8.
4. Stewart JD, et al. The Epidemiology and Clinical Features of Melioidosis in Far North Queensland: Implications for Patient Management. PLoS Negl Trop Dis 2017; 11(3): e0005411.
5. Chierakul W, et al. Melioidosis in 6 Tsunami Survivors in Southern Thailand. Clin Infect Dis 2005; 41(7): 982–90.
6. Svensson E, et al. Cutaneous Melioidosis in a Swedish Tourist after the Tsunami in 2004. Scand J Infect Dis 2006; 38(1): 71–4.
7. Thaipadungpanit J, et al. *Burkholderia pseudomallei* in Water Supplies, Southern Thailand. Emerg Infect Dis 2014; 20(11): 1947–9.
8. Hinjoy S, et al. Melioidosis in Thailand: Present and Future. Trop Med Infect Dis 2018; 3(2): 38.

9. Bhengsri S, et al. Incidence of Bacteremic Melioidosis in Eastern and Northeastern Thailand. Am J Trop Med Hyg 2011; 85(1): 117–20.

10. Trinh TT, et al. Melioidosis in Vietnam: Recently Improved Recognition but Still an Uncertain Disease Burden after Almost a Century of Reporting. Trop Med Infect Dis 2018; 3(2): 39.

11. Van Phung L, et al. Pilot Study of Exposure to *Pseudomonas pseudomallei* in Northern Vietnam. Trans R Soc Trop Med Hyg 1993; 87(4): 416.

12. Dance DAB, et al. Melioidosis in the Lao People's Democratic Republic. Trop Med Infect Dis 2018; 3(1): 21.

13. Nathan S, et al. Melioidosis in Malaysia: Incidence, Clinical Challenges, and Advances in Understanding Pathogenesis. Trop Med Infect Dis 2018; 3(1): 25.

14. Pang L, et al. Melioidosis, Singapore, 2003-2014. Emerg Infect Dis 2018; 24(1): 140–3.

15. Mukhopadhyay C, et al. Melioidosis in South Asia (India, Nepal, Pakistan, Bhutan and Afghanistan). Trop Med Infect Dis 2018; 3(2).

16. Mohapatra PR, et al. Melioidosis. Lancet Infect Dis 2019; 19(10): 1056–7.

17. Chewapreecha C, et al. Global and Regional Dissemination and Evolution of *Burkholderia pseudomallei*. Nat Microbiol 2017; 2: 16263.

18. Cheng AC, et al. Extreme Weather Events and Environmental Contamination Are Associated with Case-Clusters of Melioidosis in the Northern Territory of Australia. Int J Epidemiol 2006; 35(2): 323–9.

19. Ko WC, et al. Melioidosis Outbreak after Typhoon, Southern Taiwan. Emerg Infect Dis 2007; 13(6): 896–8.

20. Rachlin A, et al. A Cluster of Melioidosis Infections in Hatchling Saltwater Crocodiles (Crocodylus porosus) Resolved Using Genome-Wide Comparison of a Common North Australian Strain of *Burkholderia pseudomallei*. Microb Genom 2019; 5(8): e000288.

21. Currie BJ, et al. A Cluster of Melioidosis Cases from an Endemic Region Is Clonal and Is Linked to the Water Supply Using Molecular Typing of *Burkholderia pseudomallei* Isolates. Am J Trop Med Hyg 2001; 65(3): 177–9.

22. Inglis TJ, et al. Acute Melioidosis Outbreak in Western Australia. Epidemiol Infect 1999; 123(3): 437–43.

23. Limmathurotsakul D, et al. Melioidosis Caused by *Burkholderia pseudomallei* in Drinking Water, Thailand, 2012. Emerg Infect Dis 2014; 20(2): 265–8.

24. White NJ. Melioidosis. Lancet 2003; 361(9370): 1715–22.

25. Mohanty S, et al. Melioidosis of the Head and Neck: A Case Series from Eastern India. Infect Dis Rep 2020; 12(3): 36–45.

26. Ralph A, et al. Transmission of *Burkholderia pseudomallei* via Breast Milk in Northern Australia. Pediatr Infect Dis J 2004; 23(12): 1169–71.

27. Merritt AJ, et al. Cutaneous Melioidosis Cluster Caused by Contaminated Wound Irrigation Fluid. Emerg Infect Dis 2016; 22(8): 1420–7.

28. Gal D, et al. Contamination of Hand Wash Detergent Linked to Occupationally Acquired Melioidosis. Am J Trop Med Hyg 2004; 71(3): 360–2.

History of Melioidosis

3

Prasanta R Mohapatra

Department of Pulmonary Medicine and Critical Care,
All India Institute of Medical Sciences, Bhubaneswar, India

Contents

The term 'melioidosis' was first coined in 1921.[1] The name is derived from the Greek word *melis,* which means "a distemper of asses" with the suffixes -oid meaning "similar to" and -osis meaning "a condition," that is, a condition similar to glanders.[2]

The dawn of the initial concept of today's melioidosis was by pathologist Alfred Whitmore and his assistant C.S. Krishnaswami in Rangoon (renamed later as Yangon) in Myanmar (formerly Burma), as they described in their landmark paper published in 1912.[3] They first saw this malady as 'a glanders-like disease occurring in Rangoon and isolated the organism.[3] The first case was from a post-mortem examination of a 40-year-old Burman morphia addict, who succumbed after 10 days of illness. They found several abscesses at the site of his morphine injections and cheesy consolidation scattered in both lungs. The smear he prepared suggested the possibility of glanders. Krishnaswami noted the similarity to *Bacillus mallei,* but distinguished it from the new disease and suggested the name *Bacillus pseudomallei* in his 1913 paper. His paper described 38 cases (from whom the organism was isolated) were studied over 18 months but has one post-mortem case. As 31 of his 38 cases had the identification marks of morphia injections, the disease was also called 'morphia injectors' septicemia' initially by Captain

DOI: 10.1201/9781003324010-3

Knapp.[4] This septicemia series was later published by his colleague Krishnaswami.[5] Krishnaswami conducted animal experiments; the cultures of the organism were grown with success from the experimental animals' post-mortem. This was the first culture isolation of the organism. The isolation elegantly fulfilled Koch's postulates. The series was published based on their autopsy study in a report.[6] Whitmore stayed in Rangoon until 1927, becoming one of the civil surgeons and attending the family of King Thibaw on more than one occasion, serving in the Army during the First World War, rising to the rank of Lieutenant-Colonel and being instrumental in the establishment of the Burma Medical School. He continued to work on his research and teach until his death on 26 June 1946, despite undergoing major surgery in 1943.[7]

Whitmore rapidly published the clinical features of the disease. He also compared the resemblance of the disease to glanders, correlated to the infection among horses, and the possible characteristics of the micro-organism. Whitmore had also proposed the name *Bacillus pseudomallei*. The description proposed by Whitmore has been partly retained in its current nomenclature, *Burkholderia pseudomallei*. Stanton and Fletcher, after eight years, named it melioidosis.[2,6,7] Later, the taxonomic studies confirmed this, indicating that *Burkholderia mallei*, which is derived from a clone of Whitmore's *bacillus pseudomallei*, was finally named *Burkholderia pseudomallei,* the current nomenclature. Stanton and Fletcher presumed that melioidosis was a zoonosis with a reservoir in rodents and a disease infecting humans, and rodents. They coined the name 'melioidosis' for Whitmore's disease in 1921, derived from the Greek word whose meaning is a 'distemper of asses.'[2,8]

In Sri Lanka, the first human case of melioidosis was reported in 1927.[1] Later, 83 patients were reported in 1932, from the south and southeast Asia, with 98% mortality.[1,9] In 1937, the habitats of *B. pseudomallei* were established in soil and water.[1,10]

In 1949, it was found to infect sheep and goats in northern Australia by Cottew.[11] The human cases reported in Australia during 1950.[12] Recent studies have suggested that *B. pseudomallei* might have started initially in Australia and spread during the glacial period across the archipelago between mainland Indochina and Australia[13] and remained undetected during the early period.[13,14] The disease in Australia is seen most frequently in tropical regions, including among the Aboriginal communities.[15] African strains possibly originated from Asia and are also linked to the South American strains, which reflect a newer shared evolutionary history.[16] European investigators had identified the Burkholderia infection in the Dutch East Indies and French Indochina (now Cambodia, Laos, and Vietnam), where the organism was first revealed as an environmental saprophyte. The French researcher in Indochina had proved the bacteria as saprophyte rather than a zoonosis as initially assumed.[10,17] There had been quite a lot of earlier environmental work done by the French and US scientists in Malaysia on the distribution of *Pseudomonas pseudomallei* in soil and surface water.[18]

THE 'VIETNAMESE TIME BOMB'

A French scientist in Indochina (now Cambodia, Laos, and Vietnam) proved that the organism was a saprophyte rather than a zoonosis, as had initially been suspected.

It was first French soldiers; afterward, American soldiers were deployed in Vietnam and developed the disease when battle-related skin lesions were exposed to the soil and surface water that harbored *B. pseudomallei*. Helicopter staff and troops also experienced a varying load of infections. They possibly got the disease through inhaling bacteria lodged in dust and aerosols, along with a large volume of air thrashed by the helicopter's rotor fan blades.[19] Of the American soldiers and crews who were exposed to the organism, possibly by inhalation of contaminated soil dust during their stay in the endemic areas of Vietnam, a few developed the disease long after returning to place home. This disease was initially difficult to diagnose and even to find the cause in America, and when diagnosed, it was called the 'Vietnamese Time Bomb.'[20] Although such uniqueness looks imaginary, the history of crewing jobs in endemic countries is scientifically correlated to bacteria's longer latency. Although imaginary and highly unusual amongst bacterial infections, it is poorly understood.

AWARENESS IN THAILAND

Thailand was not mentioned in the history of early descriptions of melioidosis; possibly, it was never under a colonial power nor much connected externally. The first case was reported from Thailand in 1955 by Chittvej et al.[21]

Punyagupta and colleagues, during the 1980s, took an interest in creating awareness in Thailand through the Infectious Disease Association of Thailand. Such awareness control paved the way for the diagnosis of more and more cases. The actual situation gets revealed in better forms and begins to emerge. The association organized meetings and conferences from 1985 onward on the number of indigenous cases. From 1986, the Wellcome–Mahidol Oxford Tropical Medicine Research Programme supported Thailand's endeavors. Over time, Thailand emerged as one of the leaders in clinical and epidemiological research on melioidosis.[22]

From a management point of view, the year 1989 was very important. The earlier treatment for managing melioidosis was a combination of three drugs, co-trimoxazole, chloramphenicol, and doxycycline, with a very low success rate. The regimen was associated with a mortality rate of 80%.[2] In 1989, ceftazidime had shown dramatic improvement from disease and reduced the risk of death from melioidosis from 74% to 37%.[22,23] The key milestones pointing to treatment success by the dramatic reduction of mortality from melioidosis by using the antibiotic ceftazidime as a treatment during 1989.[23] In 1992, the pathogen was formally named *B. pseudomallei*.[23]

Quantitative isolation of *Burkholderia pseudomallei* from the soil in Thailand was reported in 1995.[24] In Bangladesh, the first *B. pseudomallei* was isolated from the soil of Gazipur in 2013.[25] In India, soil samples were collected from paddy fields in the coastal areas of Tamil Nādu in 2010 and confirmed by 16S rDNA sequencing.[26] Although the diseases are yet to be reported from Pakistan in the present era, despite uncertainty in methodology to distinguish *B. mallei* and *B. pseudomallei*, the published report from Pakistan has revealed the existence of *B. pseudomallei* in soil samples collected from Lahore.[27]

GENOMIC DISCOVERY

An important milestone in the history of melioidosis research was the documentation of the genome of *B. pseudomallei* in 2004, coinciding with the fourth World Melioidosis Congress in Singapore. Over the past three decades, new interest in melioidosis has been discovered and recognized around the world.[28] In 1917, about 1 in 20 post-mortems in Rangoon General Hospital revealed melioidosis, Krishnaswamy reported.[5] In 2015, *B. pseudomallei* DNA was detected from filtered air using quantitative PCR.[29] Whole-genome sequencing linked the bacteria found from home air samples at the residence of a patient with presumptive inhalational melioidosis. The study used whole-genome sequencing to link the environmental bacteria to *B. pseudomallei* recovered from the patient with mediastinal melioidosis.[30] In 2016, the global burden of human melioidosis estimation revealed 165,000 cases and 89,000 deaths yearly.[31]

BIOTHREATS

Interest and importance to melioidosis have been expressed because *Burkholderia pseudomallei* has the potential to be used as a biological weapon.[32] Though *Burkholderia pseudomallei* has not been used as a biological weapon; its close bacteria, *B. mallei*, were used by Germany against animals and infected the livestock shipped to the allied countries during the first World War and by the infamous Japanese unit in human experiments. The Japanese carried out the deliberate infection of prisoners of war and animals experimentally using *B. mallei* in China's Pingfang District during World War II.[33] It has been alleged that the Soviet Union used *B. mallei* during the Soviet-Afghan War between 1982 and 1984.[32] Ironically, probably one of the biggest ever boosts to global melioidosis research came when the US Centers for Disease Control classified *B. pseudomallei* as a 'category B' select agent.[34,35] This has facilitated American interest in the organism and disease, as well as funding for melioidosis research. This has also consequently led to an increase in the number of publications in the field.[32] *B. pseudomallei* is readily available in the environment and is cost-effective. It can also be aerosolized and transmitted via inhalation. However, the *B. pseudomallei* has never been used in biological warfare.[36]

NETWORKING

The Thailand Melioidosis Network was formed in 2012 and has been functioning closely with the Ministry of Public Health (MoPH) of Thailand. International Melioidosis Network (IMN) is a Web-based (https://www.melioidosis.info/) open network under Mahidol University, Thailand.[37] The African Melioidosis Network (AMEN) was started in 2014 with the aim of environmental and serological surveillance and capacity building of diagnostic laboratories to identify *B. pseudomallei*.[38] Many other networks, such as the Melioidosis Research Coordination Network (RCN), the Thailand Melioidosis Network (TMN), the Research Network on Melioidosis in Vietnam, the Laos Training Event for Awareness of Melioidosis (L-TEAM), the Indian Melioidosis Research Forum (IMRF), and The European Union melioidosis network have been formed to increase awareness, improve coordination, foster research collaborations, and creating clinical and epidemiological data that could provide further creative insights into how to tackle the infection and prevent melioidosis.

MILESTONES

Important years in the timeline of melioidosis are highlighted in Figure 3.1.

VACCINE DEVELOPMENT

The major hindrances in developing an effective vaccine are that The Bacteria can evade our immune system and survive in the intracellular environment. There has been phenotypic variability among virulent strains of *B. pseudomallei*.

In 2013, the Steering Group on Melioidosis Vaccine Development (SGMVD), consisting of a group of scientists, was created to accelerate the development of an effective vaccine.[39]

The experimental murine infection models indicate that specific antibody formation is key to protecting melioidosis. The evidence from the murine models and human infections in support of CD4+ T cell responses is essential for complete protection. The data strongly suggest that the production of IFNγ and IL-17A correlate with *B. pseudomallei*

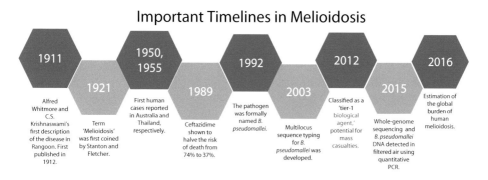

FIGURE 3.1   Timeline of Melioidosis.

deaths in mouse and human models with complete protection.[40–42] However, no recommended vaccine is available to date. Lack of immune correlates, the uncertain predictive value of animal models, and difficulty in working with *B. pseudomallei* in the laboratory have been challenges in developing a vaccine.

CONCLUSION

There has been gross under-recognition of such a mysterious disease as melioidosis in many parts of the world. The cases have been linked to global travel in the endemic regions. In a recent multi-state outbreak of melioidosis in the United States, the organism was misidentified as another bacterium, which demands the need for better diagnosis and control of the disease.[43] Despite the advancement of medical science, we have been unsuccessful over the past 11 decades in finding the actual burden of his disease amongst the underdeveloped and developing nations throughout the tropics. Melioidosis is yet to be recognized as a neglected tropical disease to improve awareness and mobilize funding for this severe and potentially fatal infectious disease.

REFERENCES

1. Wiersinga WJ, et al. Melioidosis. Nat Rev Dis Primers 2018; 4: 17107.
2. Stanton AT, et al. Melioidosis, a New Disease of the Tropics. Trans Fourth Congress Far East Assoc Trop Med, Bat 1921; 2: 196–98.
3. Whitmore A, et al. A Hitherto Undescribed Infective Disease in Rangoon. Ind Med Gaz 1912; 47(7): 262–67.
4. Knapp HHG. Morphine Injector's Septicæmia ("Whitmore's Disease"). Ind Med Gaz 1915; 50(8): 287–88.
5. Krishnaswami CS. Morphia Injectors' Septicaemia. Ind Med Gaz 1917; 52: 296–99.
6. Whitmore A. An Account of a Glanders-Like Disease Occurring in Rangoon. J Hyg (Lond) 1913; 13(1): 1–34.
7. Dance D. A Glanders-Like Disease in Rangoon: Whitmore A. J Hyg 1913; 13: 1–34. Epidemiol Infect 2005; 133(Suppl 1): S9–s10.
8. Stanton AT, et al. Two Cases of Melioidosis. J Hyg (Lond) 1924; 23(3): 268–76.
9. Stanton ATWF. Melioidosis. London, UK: John Bale and Danielson Ltd; 1932.
10. Chambon L. Isolation of Whitmore's Bacillus from External Environment. Ann Inst Pasteur (Paris) 1955; 89(2): 229–35.
11. Cottew GS. Melioidosis in Sheep in Queens Land; A Description of the Causal Organism. Aust J Exp Biol Med Sci 1950; 28(6): 677–83.
12. Rimington RA. Melioidosis in North Queensland. Med J Aust 1962; 49(1): 50–3.
13. Pearson T, et al. Phylogeographic Reconstruction of a Bacterial Species with High Levels of Lateral Gene Transfer. BMC Biol 2009; 7: 78.
14. Tuanyok A, et al. A Horizontal Gene Transfer Event Defines Two Distinct Groups within *Burkholderia Pseudomallei* That Have Dissimilar Geographic Distributions. J Bacteriol 2007; 189(24): 9044–9.

15. Cheng AC, et al. Melioidosis: Epidemiology, Pathophysiology and Management. Clin Microbiol Rev 2005; 18(2): 383–416.
16. Sarovich DS, et al. Phylogenomic Analysis Reveals an Asian Origin for African *Burkholderia Pseudomallei* and Further Supports Melioidosis Endemicity in Africa. Msphere 2016; 1(2): e00089.
17. Vaucel M. Présence probable du bacille de whitmore dans l'eau de mare au tonkin. Masson; 1937.
18. Strauss JM, et al. Melioidosis in Malaysia. II. Distribution of Pseudomonas Pseudomallei in Soil and Surface Water. Am J Trop Med Hyg 1969; 18(5): 698–702.
19. Howe C, et al. The Pseudomallei Group: A Review. J Infect Dis 1971; 124(6): 598–606.
20. Goshorn RK. Recrudescent Pulmonary Melioidosis. A Case Report Involving the So-Called 'Vietnamese Time Bomb'. Indiana Med 1987; 80(3): 247–9.
21. Chittvej C, et al. Melioidosis with Case Report in a Thai. Thai Army Med J 1955; 68: 11–17.
22. Jayanetra P, et al. Pseudomonas Pseudomallei: 1. Infection in Thailand. Southeast Asian J Trop Med Public Health 1974; 5(4): 487–91.
23. White NJ, et al. Halving of Mortality of Severe Melioidosis by Ceftazidime. Lancet 1989; 2(8665): 697–701.
24. Smith MD, et al. Quantitative Recovery of *Burkholderia Pseudomallei* from Soil in Thailand. Trans R Soc Trop Med Hyg 1995; 89(5): 488–90.
25. Chowdhury S, et al. The Epidemiology of Melioidosis and Its Association with Diabetes Mellitus: A Systematic Review and Meta-Analysis. Pathogens 2022; 11(2): 149.
26. Prakash A, et al. Isolation, Identification and Characterization of *Burkholderia Pseudomallei* from Soil of Coastal Region of India. Springerplus 2014; 3: 438.
27. Limmathurotsakul D, et al. Predicted Global Distribution of *Burkholderia Pseudomallei* and Burden of Melioidosis. Nat Microbiol 2016; 1(1): 15008.
28. Currie BJ, et al. The Global Distribution of *Burkholderia Pseudomallei* and Melioidosis: An Update. Trans R Soc Trop Med Hyg 2008; 102(Suppl 1): S1–S4.
29. Chen PS, et al. Airborne Transmission of Melioidosis to Humans from Environmental Aerosols Contaminated with *B. Pseudomallei*. PLoS Negl Trop Dis 2015; 9(6): e0003834.
30. Currie BJ, et al. Use of Whole-Genome Sequencing to Link *Burkholderia Pseudomallei* from Air Sampling to Mediastinal Melioidosis, Australia. Emerg Infect Dis 2015; 21(11): 2052–4.
31. Limmathurotsakul D, et al. Predicted Global Distribution of *Burkholderia Pseudomallei* and Burden of Melioidosis. Nat Microbiol 2016; 1(1): 15008.
32. Nguyen HN, et al. Glanders and melioidosis. In: StatPearls [Internet]. Treasure Island, FL: StatPearls Publishing; 2021.
33. Ngauy V, et al. Cutaneous Melioidosis in a Man Who Was Taken as a Prisoner of War by the Japanese During World War II. J Clin Microbiol 2005; 43(2): 970–2.
34. Rotz LD, et al. Public Health Assessment of Potential Biological Terrorism Agents. Emerg Infect Dis 2002; 8(2): 225–30.
35. Samuel M, et al. Interventions for Treating Melioidosis. Cochrane Database Syst Rev 2001; (2): Cd001263.
36. Foong YC, et al. Melioidosis: A Review. Rural Remote Health 2014; 14(4): 2763.
37. International Melioidosis Network, Microbiology department at mahidol Oxford tropical medicine research unit (MORU), Mahidol University https://www.melioidosis.info/ (accessed 06 July 2022).
38. Steinmetz I, et al. Melioidosis in Africa: Time to Uncover the True Disease Load. Trop Med Infect Dis 2018; 3(2): 62.
39. Limmathurotsakul D, et al. Consensus on the Development of Vaccines Against Naturally Acquired Melioidosis. Emerg Infect Dis 2015; 21(6): e141480.
40. Morici L, et al. Novel Multi-Component Vaccine Approaches for *Burkholderia Pseudomallei*. Clin Exp Immunol 2019; 196(2): 178–88.

41. Jenjaroen K, et al. T-Cell Responses Are Associated with Survival in Acute Melioidosis Patients. PLoS Negl Trop Dis 2015; 9(10): e0004152.
42. Khakhum N, et al. Combating the Great Mimicker: Latest Progress in the Development of *Burkholderia Pseudomallei* Vaccines. Expert Rev Vaccines 2020; 19(7): 653–60.
43. Gee JE, et al. Multistate Outbreak of Melioidosis Associated with Imported Aromatherapy Spray. N Engl J Med 2022; 386(9): 861–68.

Pathogenesis and Virulence of Melioidosis

4

Srujana Mohanty

Department of Microbiology, All India Institute of Medical Sciences, Bhubaneswar, India

Contents

INTRODUCTION

Burkholderia pseudomallei, the etiologic agent of melioidosis, exists as an environmental saprophyte in moist soils and surface waters of tropical and subtropical regions. Typical features associated with infection with this Gram-negative bacterium include its ability to cause a wide variety of manifestations ranging from localized abscesses to acute pneumonia and septicemia with high case fatality rates. Severe clinical diseases are seen in people with risk factors such as diabetes mellitus, alcoholism, renal

DOI: 10.1201/9781003324010-4

disease, and chronic pulmonary disease, along with a high propensity for recrudescence in the affected person.[1,2] As an environmental organism, many factors facilitate its persistence and survival in harsh conditions and contribute to facilitating entry and subsequent invasion of susceptible hosts.[3,4]

By nature, *B. pseudomallei* is a facultative intracellular pathogen. This behavior is the key to disease pathogenesis as it can invade and replicate inside various human cells, such as polymorphonuclear leukocytes, macrophages, and epithelial cell lines. Moreover, a large 7.2 Mb genome confers the added advantage of encoding for numerous virulence factors (Table 4.1), which aid the organism in various ways.[1,5]

Disease pathogenesis often follows a defined sequence of events (Table 4.2), with the outcome and manifestations depending on a fine interplay of many organism-associated and host-associated factors. In particular, possessing a remarkable array of intrinsic virulence factors aids the organism in maintaining a survival advantage. On the other hand, the level of an intact immune system seems to be the major host-associated driving factor likely to influence disease severity and outcome.

TABLE 4.1   Selected virulence factors of *B. pseudomallei*

VIRULENCE FACTOR	FUNCTION
Surface polysaccharides: • capsular polysaccharide • lipopolysaccharide	• Inhibit opsonophagocytosis • Confer serum resistance and resistance to killing by host complement • Contribute to initial biofilm deposition • Facilitate attachment to human pharyngeal epithelial cells
Specialized secretion systems: • Cluster-3 type III • Cluster-1 type VI	• Facilitate intracellular invasion, optimal survival, and growth of the organism within host cells • Invasion of non-phagocytic cells • Rapid escape from endocytic vacuoles
Adhesins (PilA, BoaA, BoaB), flagella	• Mediate attachment to non-phagocytic cells
Secreted proteins and exoproducts: • Proteases • Lipases • Phospholipases	• Extracellular proteolytic activity
Secondary metabolites: malleipeptins and syrbactins	• Function as biosurfactants observed to be critical for virulence in BALB/c mice
Quorum sensing	• Facilitates activation of virulence factors based on environmental cues and bacterial cross-talk • Aids in widespread dissemination to different body parts
Morphotype switching	• Associated with variation in colonial morphology, such as formation of small-colony variants

TABLE 4.2   The sequence of events in *B. pseudomallei* disease pathogenesis

- Host cell attachment and cell invasion
- Intracellular survival and replication
- Intercellular spread
- Formation of multi-nucleated giant cells
- Evasion of autophagy and cell lysis
- Secondary spread
- Host response

HOST CELL ATTACHMENT AND INTRACELLULAR INVASION

Depending on the route of entry, the organism first enters and replicates in epithelial cells of the mucosal surface or broken skin and then spreads to various cell types. Entry is facilitated by various adhesins such as polar flagella, Type 4 pili, and a thin polysaccharide layer around the bacteria.[2] In non-phagocytic cells, PilA and two T5SS adhesion proteins (BoaA and BoaB) are essential for uptake, while in phagocytic cells, activation of pattern recognition receptors, such as Toll-like receptors (TLRs), which recognize conserved pathogen-associated molecular patterns (PAMPs), play an active role.[1,2]

Following attachment and uptake, intracellular invasion with subsequent survival is crucial in the pathogenesis process. Principal virulence factors that aid the bacterium to evade host defenses and replicate in the cells are the multiple secretion systems. These evolutionary apparatuses enable the transport of proteins across cellular membranes in response to the environment.[2,5] The secretion systems are classified considering their structure, function, and specificity. The type III secretion system (T3SS) expression, which is triggered upon bacterial contact with the host cell following adhesin-mediated attachment, functions like a molecular syringe. Permeating through the inner and outer bacterial cell membranes, the T3SS forms a filamentous needle-like projection through which the bacteria can translocate effector proteins from its cytoplasm into host cells via a pore created in the host cell membrane by these proteins. Subsequently, intracellular invasion, survival, and growth of *B. pseudomallei* are largely aided by the type III secretion system cluster 3 (T3SS-3) and type VI secretion system cluster 1 (T6SS-1). Effector proteins of T3SS that have an important role, include the *Burkholderia* invasion proteins (Bip), namely BipB, -C, and -D.[5,6] Some other proteins aid in the process, namely, BopA, BopE and BsaQ. BopE (a guanine nucleotide exchange factor) causes rearrangement of the host actin cytoskeleton (membrane ruffling) and facilitates ingress.[1]

Host factors also play a part in epithelial attachment. Protease-activated receptor 1 (PAR1, which belongs to the subfamily of G protein-coupled receptors) is expressed on several cell types (for example, endothelial cells, platelets, and monocytes) and promotes *B. pseudomallei* cell invasion, growth, and dissemination.

INTRACELLULAR SURVIVAL AND REPLICATION

Following endocytosis, survival within the endocytic vesicles is facilitated by the production of a protease inhibitor, ecotin, which resists degradation by lysosomal enzymes.[1,2] Next, the bacteria escape from the primary endosome via T3SS, replicates in the cytosol, and proceeds to localize in the nuclei of infected cells, with a potential for intracellular persistence in this location.

SURVIVAL WITHIN MACROPHAGES

B. pseudomallei has the ability to multiply within phagocytic cells (macrophages, monocytes, neutrophils) without profound activation of a bactericidal response, even when lysosomal fusion occurs. An important mechanism of cell killing effected by phagocytes to control intracellular replication is mediated by reactive nitrogen intermediates and reactive oxygen species (superoxide ions and H_2O_2) produced as a result of the action of inducible nitric oxide synthase (iNOS) enzyme. Evolutionarily, *B. pseudomallei* has developed mechanisms to suppress the iNOS production by activating two negative regulatory cytokines: suppressor of cytokine signaling 3 (SOCS3) and cytokine-inducible SH2- containing protein (CIS), thus protecting itself from the phagocyte-mediated killing.[5,6] In addition, degrading enzymes that inactivate reactive oxygen species and ability to delay polymorphonuclear apoptosis favor bacterial survival.

INTERCELLULAR SPREAD

As the bacteria becomes free in the host cell cytosol due to escape from the phagosomes, it induces host actin polymerization and propels itself throughout the cell. Subsequently, it spreads to neighboring cells by either actin- or flagellum (*fla2*)-mediated motility aided by cell fusion. An important virulence gene facilitating such intercellular spread is the *bimA*, the functional BimA protein being involved in actin polymerization, with *bimA* mutants unable to form actin tails.[1,2,6] In addition, type VI secretion system cluster 5 (T6SS-5) and two other genes of the T6SS complex, namely, *hcp* and *vgrG* genes demonstrate a significant role in both intercellular spread and virulence.[1,5,6] Hcp creates tubules that facilitate protein translocation across the membranes of host cells. Valine-glycine repeat protein (VgrG) is required for cell fusion and, therefore, intercellular organism spread.

FORMATION OF MULTI-NUCLEATED GIANT CELLS

The ability of *B. pseudomallei* and related species to stimulate host cell fusion results in the formation of multi-nucleated giant cells (MNGC), which further promote localized dissemination and immune system escape. In addition to T6SS, other virulence factors involved in the successful formation of MNGC, include expression of the gene *lfpA* and functional T3SS-3.[2,6]

EVASION OF AUTOPHAGY AND CELL LYSIS

This process mediated by T3SS-dependent effector protein BopA involves the activation of nucleotide-binding oligomerization domain-containing protein 2 (NOD2, an intracellular pathogen recognition receptor), resulting in bacterial killing.[1,2] However, the complete mechanisms of autophagy escape are yet to be elucidated. Macrophage lysis could represent an escape mechanism for *B. pseudomallei* once a threshold bacterial load has been reached.

SECONDARY SPREAD

Bacteremic dissemination to a variety of sites from a primary focus of respiratory melioidosis is principally mediated by capsular polysaccharide, which impairs opsonization, reduces complement efficacy, and enables organism persistence in the blood, resulting in the increased ability to infect end organs. Profound dissemination is also aided by lipopolysaccharide, flagella, pili, quorum sensing, T3SS, T6SS, and morphotype switching.[2,5]

SMALL COLONY VARIANTS

One of the resultant effects of morphotype switching is the formation of small colony variants, which often have reduced susceptibility to antibiotics and an enhanced ability to cause latent or recurrent infection.[2] Certain colony variants, such as yellow colony variant B, are capable of survival in the stomach environment, with some others showing increased cellular adherence.

HOST RESPONSE

Disease outcomes, whether asymptomatic, acute, chronic, or latent disease are likely determined by host response to a large extent. An exaggerated host immune response with hyperproduction of proinflammatory cytokines can result in tissue destruction and organ failure. Neutrophils have a key role in host response as they can kill up to 90% of intracellular organisms, eliminate extracellular bacteria via neutrophil extracellular traps, and are able to promote generation of the host cytokine response. Significantly, as all these neutrophil phagocytic functions are likely to be reduced in patients with poor glycemic control with other underlying co-morbidities; in older patients, the chances of severity also increase proportionately in these population groups. In addition to the neutrophil-mediated innate immunity, a robust cell-mediated immunity also appears to be essential for halting the progression of the disease. Poor clinical outcomes observed in severe bacteremic melioidosis are associated with high levels of proinflammatory cytokines, IFN-γ, interleukin 6 (IL-6), and IL-18.[3,4]

The current literature suggests that acute melioidosis results from a combinatorial interplay of ineffective innate cellular immune responses with both the critical role of antibodies and Th1-adaptive responses being necessary for the successful prevention/ eradication of melioidosis. However, in all likelihood, a substantial number of as yet unknown pathogen-associated, host-associated, and environment-associated genes still remain to be explored for a full understanding of the pathogenetic process of this elusive bacterium.

REFERENCES

1. Stone JK, DeShazer D, Brett PJ, Burtnick MN. Melioidosis: Molecular Aspects of Pathogenesis. Expert Rev Anti Infect Ther. 2014 Dec;12(12):1487–99. doi: 10.1586/14787210. 2014.970634.
2. Gassiep I, Armstrong M, Norton R. Human Melioidosis. Clin Microbiol Rev. 2020 Mar 11;33(2): e00006–19. doi: 10.1128/CMR.00006-19.
3. Currie BJ. Melioidosis: Evolving Concepts in Epidemiology, Pathogenesis, and Treatment. Semin Respir Crit Care Med. 2015 Feb;36(1):111–25. doi: 10.1055/s-0034-1398389.
4. Wiersinga WJ, Currie BJ, Peacock SJ. Melioidosis. N Engl J Med. 2012 Sep 13;367(11): 1035–44. doi: 10.1056/NEJMra1204699.
5. Wiersinga WJ, Virk HS, Torres AG, Currie BJ, Peacock SJ, Dance DAB, Limmathurotsakul D. Melioidosis. Nat Rev Dis Primers. 2018 Feb 1;4:17107. doi: 10.1038/nrdp.2017.107.
6. Mariappan V, Vellasamy KM, Barathan M, Girija ASS, Shankar EM, Vadivelu J. Hijacking of the Host's Immune Surveillance Radars by *Burkholderia Pseudomallei*. Front Immunol. 2021 Aug 11;12:718719. doi: 10.3389/fimmu.2021.718719.

Laboratory Diagnosis of Human Melioidosis

5

Bijayini Behera

*Department of Microbiology, All India Institute
of Medical Sciences, Bhubaneswar, India*

Contents

The clinical spectrum of the melioidosis disease complex encompassing acute, rapidly progressing bacteremic infection with or without underlying focus to chronic, persistent, localized infections, and reactivation of latent disease to dormant seroconversion is an unchartered territory for clinicians without a specific laboratory diagnosis.[1] The lack of pathognomonic clinical features with elusive symptoms confounds initial diagnostic assessment, and subsequent delay in appropriate therapy significantly affects morbidity and mortality. The presence of classical/traditional risk factors such as poor glycaemic control in diabetes mellitus, heavy alcohol consumption, chronic kidney and lung diseases; putative risk factors such as cancer chemotherapy, long-term steroid/other immunosuppressive medications; cardiac diseases such as rheumatic heart disease, congestive heart failure, chronic granulomatous disease; iron overload conditions like thalassemia and pulmonary hemosiderosis, history of kava consumption, and tuberculosis increases

DOI: 10.1201/9781003324010-5

the weight of clinical suspicion of melioidosis. It helps in the optimization of initial diagnostic stewardship practices.[1] Melioidosis should be included in the differentials in the following conditions, particularly in endemic areas.

1. Prolonged fever (>3 weeks) not responding to conventional antimicrobials without an immediately apparent etiology, especially during the rainy season.
2. Presence of acute onset community-acquired sepsis, defined as presence of two or more of the following, i.e., temperature <36°C or >38°C, tachycardia (Heart rate >90 beats/minute), tachypnoea (respiratory rate >20/minute), total white cell count of <4,000 or >12,000 cells/mm^3 or band forms >10%.[2]
3. Presence of acute onset community-acquired pneumonia presenting with cough, purulent expectoration, shortness of breath and/or pleuritic chest pain with variable radiological features (e.g., minimal infiltrates/cavitation/diffuse parenchymal disease) and not responding to conventional antimicrobials (e.g., standard dosing regimens of β lactams, macrolides, or fluoroquinolones).
4. Parenchymal visceral abscesses (e.g., spleen, liver, kidney) with characteristic ultrasonographic features (Swiss cheese appearance of tiny, dispersed abscesses). Intracerebral abscesses, prostatic abscesses, and parotid abscesses (especially in children).
5. Chronic ulcerative/pustular cutaneous lesions, unresponsive to conventional antimicrobials.
6. Fever, weight loss, and productive cough with predominantly upper lobe infiltrates on chest radiography mimicking pulmonary tuberculosis.
7. Lymphadenitis, particularly involving the cervical lymph nodes.
8. Neuromelioidosis presenting with various combinations of cranial nerve palsies, cerebellar signs, and peripheral weakness.
9. Rare presentations of pyogenic lesions, including thyroid and scrotal abscesses, chronic osteomyelitis, and septic arthritis.

MICROBIOLOGICAL DIAGNOSIS

There are limitations and pitfalls in clinical and radiographic diagnosis, so microbiological diagnosis remains the cornerstone of diagnosis for the initiation of specific antimicrobial therapy. Microbiological diagnosis can be broadly classified as culture-based diagnosis (reference method) and non-culture diagnostic methods like antibody detection, direct pathogen detection in clinical specimens by immunofluorescence assay, lateral flow immunoassay, and nucleic acid amplification tests. Analysis of gene expression signatures by microarray and metabolic profiling for novel biomarkers identification are promising tools for the future.[3,4] B. pseudomallei is included in the lists of hazard group 3 pathogens and tier 1 select agents; hence appropriate safety precautions need to be followed during specimen collection, transportation, the performance of culture/non-culture-based tests, as well as during disposal of laboratory wastes as a preventive measure against laboratory-acquired melioidosis. Handling of propagative works should be ideally performed inside a class II biological safety cabinet (BSC).[5] A recent study, however, has determined the risk of developing laboratory-acquired melioidosis to be very low in settings where open bench propagative works are performed, familiar to all low and middle-income countries.[6] However, local regulations and legislation regarding handling *Burkholderia pseudomallei* should be followed.

CULTURE-BASED DIAGNOSIS

Culture is regarded as the mainstay of microbiological diagnosis, with an estimated sensitivity of approximately 60% derived from a statistical model.[7] A combination of blood, throat swab/sputum, and centrifuged urine deposit cultures are recommended to be performed on all cases of suspected melioidosis, regardless of presenting symptoms.[8] Additionally, clinical specimens such as pus, exudate, and USG-guided aspirates from deep-seated abscesses and lymph node aspirates are to be cultured depending upon the presenting symptoms. Routine procedures for collection, transport, and storage of samples for microbiological testing are usually sufficient for the isolation of *B. pseudomallei*. Routine bacteriological culture media (e.g., 5% sheep blood agar, MacConkey agar) support the growth of *B. pseudomallei*. In clinical specimens likely to be contaminated with commensal flora (e.g. sputum, throat swab, and urine), the initial enrichment culture in Ashdown broth containing colistin, followed by plating onto selective media, has been shown to increase the case detection of melioidosis by 1.6% in non-blood clinical specimens.[9] In clinical specimens expected to be contaminated with normal flora, several selective media such as Ashdown agar, *Burkholderia pseudomallei* selective agar (BPSA), and *Burkholderia cepacia* selective agar (BCSA) are used, with additional colistin and gentamicin supplements, making use of the intrinsic resistance of *B. pseudomallei* to these antimicrobials. The use of selective media for culturing clinical specimens with normal flora has been shown to establish a diagnosis of 16–20% of all melioidosis cases with minimal cost increase.[10]

   B. pseudomallei is relatively slow-growing; therefore, an incubation period of at least five days at 37°C is recommended before discarding the culture plates.[4] *B. pseudomallei* produces colonies with unique morphological characteristics on various culture media (Figure 5.1a, b, & c). On sheep blood agar, *B. pseudomallei* colonies are typically small, smooth, cream-colored with a metallic sheen, and dryness with wrinkling becoming pronounced after 48–72 hours of incubation. On MacConkey agar, colonies are initially lactose non-fermenting and opaque with a metallic sheen but assume a rugose appearance with central umbonation after 48–72 hours. On Ashdown's agar, colonies are typically pinpointed at 18 hours and evolve into a purple, flat, dry, wrinkled appearance at 48–72 hours of incubation. Extensive characterization of clinical isolates in Thailand has led to the identification of seven distinct *B. pseudomallei* colony

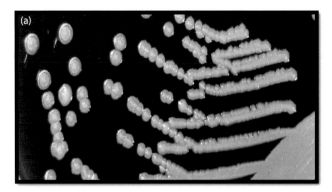

FIGURE 5.1A   Blood agar showing cream-coloured colonies with a metallic sheen.

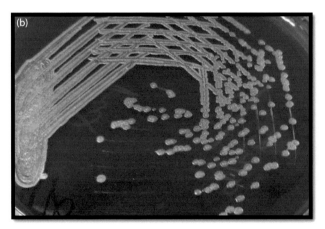

FIGURE 5.1B   MacConkey agar showing pale dry colonies with a metallic sheen and central umbonation.

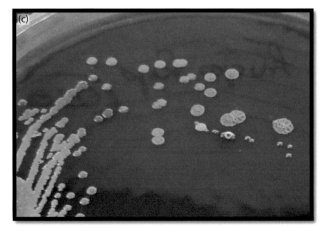

FIGURE 5.1C   Ashdown agar showing flat, dry pink colonies.

morphotypes, with type I being the most common morphotype.[11] Type III and VI morphotypes produce smooth colonies.[11]

Identification of *B. Pseudomallei* Isolates Grown on Culture

Species-level identification of *B. pseudomallei* from culture plates/broth can be ascertained by various methods such as:

Conventional biochemical tests with triple-disc screening.
Automated bacterial identification systems.
Immunoassays.
Molecular identification by polymerase chain reaction (PCR) using *B. pseudomallei*-specific primers.
Mass spectrometry.

Conventional biochemical tests with triple-disc screening

As misidentification of *B. pseudomallei* with other non-fermenters is common, several manual key identifying features (e.g., oxidase-positive, indole-negative reactions, absence of haemolysis on sheep blood agar, absence of violet pigment, irregular or bipolar morphology [safety pin appearance] on Gram staining, (Figure 5.2) triple-disc screening, e.g., susceptibility to amoxicillin-clavulanic acid [zone of inhibition measuring ≥18 mm around a 20/10 µg amoxicillin-clavulanic acid disk] and resistance to colistin or polymyxin B and gentamicin [no zone of inhibition around 10 µg colistin or polymyxin

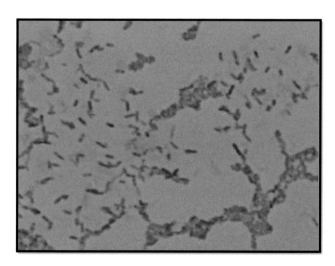

FIGURE 5.2   Gram stain showing Gram-negative bacilli with bipolar staining ('safety pin appearance').

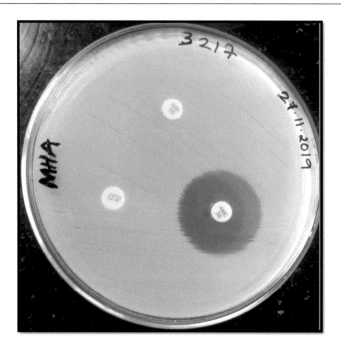

FIGURE 5.3 Presumptive identification of the *B. pseudomallei* isolate using the triple-disc test. Sensitive to amoxicillin clavulanate 30 µg, resistant to colistin 10 µg and gentamicin 10 µg.

B 300-unit disk and gentamicin 10 µg] are used in combination for species-level identification (Figure 5.3).[12] Approximately 86% of clinical *B. pseudomallei* isolates from Sarawak, Malaysia were susceptible to gentamicin in stark contrast to less than 1 in 1000 isolates in Thailand.[13,14]

Automated bacterial identification systems

Commercially available automated biochemical identification systems such as Vitek 2 (bioMérieux, France) and the Phoenix and BBL Crystal systems (Becton Dickinson, United States) are increasingly being used in diagnostic microbiology laboratories. A wide range of variations is reported in the species-level identification of *B. pseudomallei* by these systems from different endemic countries.[15,16]

In a study that evaluated the Vitek 2 colorimetric GN card, 19–98% and 53–88% of *B. pseudomallei* isolates were correctly identified in Australia and Malaysia, respectively.[15,16]

Immunoassays

Latex agglutination assays based on monoclonal antibodies targeting *B. pseudomallei*-specific lipopolysaccharide or exopolysaccharide possess excellent sensitivity (95–100%) and specificity (up to 100%) for the identification of *B. pseudomallei* isolates grown on culture.[17] It can also be performed directly from blood culture broths. It is also shown to distinguish between *B. pseudomallei* and its closely related species *Burkholderia thailandensis*. A recent development in the field of latex agglutination is the development of prototype Recombinant 94TF Bacteriophage Tail Fibre-Based assay, which has employed recombinant *Burkholderia* phage tail fiber 94 TF conjugated to latex beads.[18] The test can be performed in less than 5 minutes. It demonstrated 98% diagnostic sensitivity and specificity of 82.7% in a single-centre study from Thailand.[18] Indirect immunofluorescence microscopy is also used for the identification of *B. pseudomallei* isolates grown on culture. This requires considerable technical expertise and fluorescence microscopy facilities that are not widely used.[19]

Colony identification by PCR using B. pseudomallei-*specific primers*

Several gene targets are used in a conventional polymerase chain reaction (PCR) and real-time PCR format to confirm presumptive *B. pseudomallei* grown on culture. Most conventional PCR methods have used the 16S rDNA and type III secretion system 1 (TTS1) gene cluster as targets.[20] The discriminatory power of 16S rDNA locus in distinguishing *B. pseudomallei* from closely related *Burkholderia* species is poor, particularly *B. thailandensis*[20] because of closely related genomes (≤1% difference in the 16S ribosomal DNA gene sequences of *B. pseudomallei* and *B. thailandensis*). The type III secretion system (TTS) is a toxin delivery multi-protein assembly mechanism encoded by the core genome of *B. pseudomallei*. Analysis of core genome sequencing data had revealed the presence of two clusters of TTS genes (TTS1 and TTS2) in *B. pseudomallei*. The TTS1 gene cluster is exclusive to *B. pseudomallei* and is absent in *B. thailandensis* or *B. mallei*. The TTS2 gene cluster, on the other hand, is present in both *B. mallei* (99% identity) and *B. thailandensis*, making TTS1 a more desirable target for the identification of *B. pseudomallei*.[21] A conventional PCR-based assay designed to target *B. pseudomallei* open reading frame 2 (*orf2*) of the type III secretion system 1 (TTS1) is being considered the reference method for confirmation of presumptive *B. pseudomallei* grown on culture (Figure 5.4).[3] Several other conventional PCR use targets other than TTS1 such as *groEL*, *bdhA*, *phaC*, and *mpr*A. Similarly, various real-time PCR protocols targeting lpxO, 16s rDNA, fliC, and TTS1 are used in reference laboratories for confirmation of presumptive *B. pseudomallei* grown on culture.[20] Whole genome sequencing assists both in accurate identification as well as molecular epidemiological analysis.[22]

Mass spectrometry

Matrix-assisted laser desorption/ionization time-of-flight mass spectrometry (MALDI-TOF MS) offers a unique advantage of pathogen identification within minutes. *B. pseudomallei* is not included in the *in vitro* diagnostic use (IVD) database and is part of research use only (RUO) databases of two commercially available MS systems (MALDI Biotyper, Bruker Daltonik GmbH, and the Vitek MS BioMérieux). A multi-country evaluation of the *B. pseudomallei* spectrum using combinations of reference as well

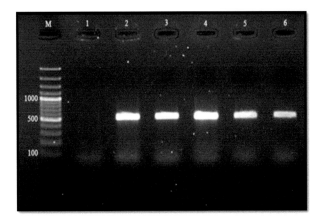

FIGURE 5.4   PCR amplified product of TTS1 Gene. **Lane M**: 100 bp ladder (ThermoFisher Scientific); **Lanes 2–6**: Presence of TTS1 gene (548 bp); **Lane 1**: Absence of TTS1 gene.

as clinical isolates achieved 100% identification of Australian as well as Asian isolates with perfect discrimination from closely related *Burkholderia thailandensis* and members of the *B. cepacia* complex (BCC) in the Vitek MS system.[23]

NON-CULTURE METHODS

Detection of *B. pseudomallei*-specific antibodies

Several assays are available to detect *B. pseudomallei*-specific antibodies, including indirect hemagglutination assay (IHA), enzyme-linked immunosorbent assay (ELISA), immunofluorescent assay, rapid immunochromatographic test, and recently, protein microarray approach. IHA is one of the oldest serological tests used for measuring humoral antibody response to *B. pseudomallei*. The test is not commercially available and requires in-house preparation and standardization of the antigen. IHA has limited utility as a diagnostic test and is mainly used in the serological survey for evidence of exposure in healthy populations residing in an endemic area; however, some endemic countries such as Australia and Sri Lanka use IHA as an adjunct diagnostic test for clinical diagnosis of melioidosis. The role of IHA in the diagnosis of this disease depends on many factors, particularly the background seropositivity in the general population as well as types of clinical presentation and patient comorbidities.[24]

A study from the northern Australian territories has demonstrated that in patients presenting with acute culture-confirmed melioidosis, IHA positivity was only

60%. On further analysis, various factors like female gender, presenting with pneumonia, and underlying chronic renal disease were found to be associated with an initially negative IHA.[25]

For the use of IHA as a diagnostic test, titres of 1:20, 1:40 or 1:80, 1:160 to 1:1280, and >1:1,280 are recommended as negative, low positive, high positive, and very high positive, respectively, in northern Australia.[25] In Sri Lanka, a single raised IHA titre of >1:1280 is regarded as positive.[26]

Few ELISAs detecting IgM and IgG have been developed and used for the serodiagnosis of melioidosis. Most of these ELISAs are home-brewed ELISAs, and the most commonly coated antigens are whole crude cell, bacterial lipopolysaccharide (LPS), exopolysaccharide (EPS), antibody affinity-purified EPS, recombinant flagellin protein, and hemolysin-coregulated protein (Hcp1).[3] Sensitivity and specificity were in the range of 72–96% for the affinity-purified EPS ELISA in a few studies from Thailand.[27] Purified O-polysaccharide (OPS) and Hcp1 are shown as potential targets for serodiagnosis of acute melioidosis in endemic areas.[28]

An immunofluorescent assay (IFAT) using whole-cell antigen for the detection of total antibodies to *B. pseudomallei* was found to be useful in monitoring the progression of the disease during maintenance therapy, apart from demonstrating good correlation in culture-positive melioidosis.[29]

Antibodies directed against Hcp1 are also detected in an immunochromatographic (ICT) format. A study evaluated the Hcp1 ICT taking culture results as the gold standard, the sensitivity was 88.3%, and the specificities ranged from 86.1% and 100%.[30]

The ICT Melioidosis Rapid Cassette Test IgG and IgM from PanBio (Windsor, Queensland, Australia) was evaluated by one Australian and one Thai study.[27] The IgG test had higher specificity (90%) and lower sensitivity (70%) compared to the IgM test, which had higher sensitivity (100%) and lower specificity (69%).[25] The clinical significance of IgM and IgG antibody responses in diagnosing melioidosis remains unclear.

A protein microarray containing 20 recombinant and purified *B. pseudomallei* proteins in a 96-well format was demonstrated to have 86.7% sensitivity and 97% specificity in a single-centre study. The assay requires further large-scale validation for the evaluation of clinical utility.[31]

Detection of B. pseudomallei-*specific antigens*

Antigen detection tests using latex agglutination tests, lateral flow immunoassay, and direct immunofluorescence tests from various specimens (such as blood, sputum, urine, or pus) have been attempted.[27] These tests have great potential to be used as a point of care tests to shorten the turnaround time for melioidosis. There is considerable variation according to the type of sample tested, which reflects different bacterial loads in different types of samples. An in-house developed latex agglutination assay targeting 200 kDa surface antigen of *B. pseudomallei* was reported to have sensitivity and specificity of

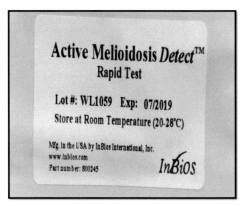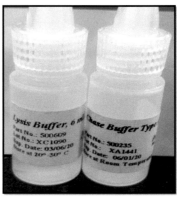

FIGURE 5.5   AMD-LFI kit with reagents (InBios, United States).

95.1% and 99.7%, respectively, in the turbid blood culture broth.[32] Direct immunofluorescence tests have a limited sensitivity of 63.7% but excellent specificity of 99.4% in samples other than blood.[27] A lateral flow immunoassay (LFI) detecting *B. pseudomallei*-specific capsular polysaccharide (CPS) was developed by InBios (Seattle, WA, United States) in the name of Active Melioidosis Detect (AMD) as a research-only use test (Figure 5.5). LFI has enormous potential to reduce the time to diagnosis of melioidosis, results are easy to interpret, and it is a field-deployable point of care test (Figure 5.6). LFI has been evaluated in several endemic countries from various samples. Overall, the serum sample demonstrates the lowest sensitivity at 27%, and sensitivities from other non-blood samples such as urine, pus, and sputum are reported to be 63%, 83%, and 85%, respectively. Urine is demonstrated to be a preferable matrix compared to serum, with a sensitivity of 40.5% and 6.5%, respectively, in a recent study.[33]Sensitivity from the serum sample was higher in bacteremic (39%) and septicaemic melioidosis with shock (68%).[34] Using multiple samples from the same patient for LFI raised the sensitivity to 91% (21/23) in one study from Odisha, India.[35] Original versions of AMD had limitations of producing non-specific bands in urine samples from non-melioidosis patients. To overcome this limitation, the manufacturers have developed a new version of the assay AMD plus with an inhibitory agent.[34] Recent findings from a single-centre study also suggest heating of pus and sputum samples prior to LFI increases sensitivity; however it needs validation across large-scale multi-centric studies.[34] A recent cohort-based case-control study in Thailand showed combinations of LFI detecting *B. pseudomallei*-specific CPS antigen in combination with OPS and Hcp1 antibody ELISAs had improved sensitivities in the diagnosis of melioidosis, compared to antigen

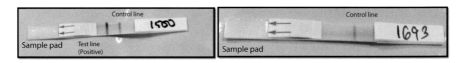

FIGURE 5.6   AMD-LFI strip showing a positive test (left) and a negative test result (right).

testing and antibody testing alone.[36] *B. pseudomallei* capsular polysaccharide antigen is included in a multiplex lateral flow immunoassay format (DPP® Fever Panel II Asia) for the diagnosis of pathogens that commonly cause febrile illness in Southeast Asia. A recent cohort-based case-control study of (DPP® Fever Panel II Asia) in Thailand found a sensitivity of 27% for diagnosis of melioidosis.[37]

Molecular detection of B. pseudomallei directly from clinical specimens

Molecular methods employed for the detection of *B. pseudomallei* in clinical samples include conventional gel PCR as well as quantitative real-time PCR (qPCR)-based methodologies or isothermal technologies such as LAMP and recombinase polymerase amplification assay. Several targets such as 16s r RNA, 16s-23s r RNA ITS, fliC, rps U, TTS1 orf2, TTS1 orf11, TTS1 orfD, lpxO, mpr A, 8653, 9438, 266152 targeting the methyl malonate-semialdehyde dehydrogenase gene locus, Tat domain, YLF/BTFC, and psu, pkku-s23-LPS have been evaluated in conventional PCR and/or (qPCR) format from a variety of clinical specimens.[38] A PCR assay targeting TTS1-orf 2 of *B. pseudomallei* has been shown to be the most reliable assay. It has been evaluated in both conventional as well as a real-time format for the diagnosis of melioidosis. qPCR targeting the type III secretion system (TTS 1) gene is reported to have an overall sensitivity of 75% in septicaemic melioidosis.[39] Sensitivity of TTS1-orf 2 conventional PCR ranged from 28% in serum to 100% in sputum and wound swab, with an overall sensitivity of 77% in septicaemic melioidosis cases.[40]

Isothermal amplification technologies such as LAMP and RPA are cheaper alternatives to PCR but have been evaluated by very few studies. A single study evaluating LAMP for the diagnosis of melioidosis reported a very low sensitivity of 30.2%, though specificity was 98.5%.[41]

RPA-LFA was evaluated in a few studies in comparison qPCR to evaluate the limit of detection in artificially spiked samples. RPA- LFA performs better in whole blood samples, showing less interference by inhibitors. Primer design and limited manufacturing of consumables are the biggest hindrances to the widespread application of RPA techniques.[42,43]

NOVEL METHODS

To overcome the shortcomings of using LFI in whole blood samples, a novel i-STAT device employing anti-CPS monoclonal antibodies has been developed. The i-STAT assay demonstrated 76% sensitivity and 94% specificity from blood specimens. Additionally, it could detect 32% of blood culture-negative melioidosis patients.[44]

Host gene expression signatures obtained from microarray data are being explored for early diagnosis of melioidosis with two differentially expressed genes, *AIM2* (absent in melanoma 2) and *FAM26F* (family with sequence similarity 26, member F) being evaluated for the early diagnosis of melioidosis.[4] Metabolomics is also being studied for the identification of novel biomarkers.[3]

A step-wise diagnostic approach is depicted to optimize the laboratory diagnosis in resource-limited settings (Flow Chart below).

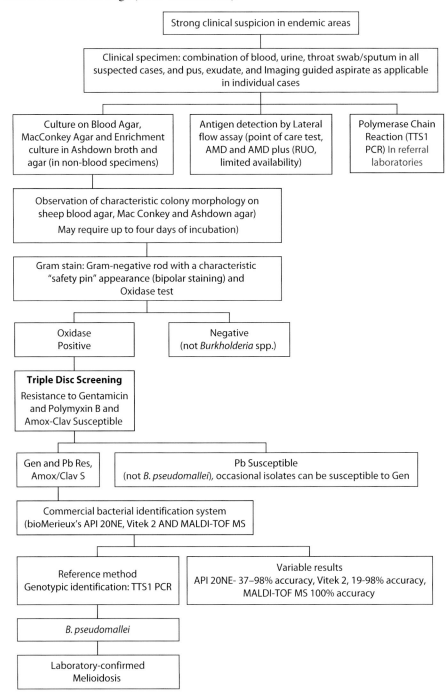

ANTIMICROBIAL SUSCEPTIBILITY TESTING

Melioidosis has limited therapeutic options, and treatment is divided into an early intensive and prolonged eradication phase. The administration of antibiotics, to which *B. pseudomallei* isolates are resistant, can have serious consequences on patient outcomes; hence, it is necessary to perform routine antimicrobial susceptibility tests.

Although antimicrobial resistance in clinical *B. pseudomallei* isolates is relatively rare, resistance emergence may compromise therapeutic efficacies. It is necessary to perform routine antimicrobial susceptibility tests to monitor trends. The Clinical and Laboratory Standards Institute (CLSI) recommends minimum inhibitory concentration (MIC) testing by the broth microdilution method.[45] However, interpretative standards for zone sizes by disk diffusion testing have been provided by the British Society of Antimicrobial Chemotherapy (BSAC), UK, and recently by EUCAST.[46] The disk diffusion and MIC breakpoints are tabulated in Table 5.1. Zone diameter (EUCAST) and MIC breakpoints for Burkholderia pseudomallei (CLSI M45) are given in Table 5.1.

As per EUCAST, ceftazidime and co-trimoxazole can be prescribed even if the isolates are labeled as I (susceptible, increased exposure).[47]

There are reports of the overcalling of co-trimoxazole resistance by the disc diffusion method; hence, isolates should be reported as resistant only by MIC-based methods.[48]

TABLE 5.1 Zone Diameter and Mic Breakpoints for *Burkholderia pseudomallei*

ANTIMICROBIAL AGENT	DISK CONTENT (μg)	EUCAST INTERPRETATIVE CATEGORIES AND ZONE DIAMETER BREAKPOINTS (mm)			CLSI INTERPRETATIVE CATEGORIES AND MIC BREAKPOINTS (μg/ml)		
		S≥	I	R<	S≤	I	R≥
Ceftazidime	10	50	18–49	18	8	16	32
Trimethoprim-sulfamethoxazole	1.25–23.75	50	17–49	17	2/38	–	4/76
Imipenem	10	29	N/A	29	4	8	16
Meropenem	10	24	N/A	24	–	–	–
Amoxicillin-clavulanate	20–10	50	22–49	22	8/4	16/8	32/16
Doxycycline	30	–	–	–	4	8	16
Chloramphenicol	30	50	22–49	22	–	–	–

Note: N/A: Not Applicable

CONCLUSION

Culture remains the gold standard for microbial diagnosis and should be attempted wherever possible for the definitive diagnosis of melioidosis. The use of a combination of samples like blood, sputum/throat swab, urine, and pus/aspirate, as well as the use of enrichment and selective culture media for respiratory samples from suspected cases of melioidosis have been shown to increase the diagnostic yield of culture. It is equally important to culture specimens from deep-seated clinical foci of infection, assisted by imaging studies wherever possible. Increased awareness is necessary among microbiologists to avoid misidentification of *Burkholderia pseudomallei* as *Pseudomonas* spp or disregarding growth as possible contaminants. Molecular assay targeting type III secretion system I (TTS1) by conventional or a real-time PCR platform is considered the reference method for species-level identification and differentiation from closely related *Burkholderia* spp. Point-of-care tests that detect capsular polysaccharide antigens (InBios Active Melioidosis Detect lateral flow test, for research only use) must be validated in large-scale multi-centric studies. Currently available serodiagnosis methods alone cannot be relied on to make a definitive diagnosis of melioidosis due to suboptimal sensitivity, specificity, and a lack of international standardization. The deployment of molecular assay directly from clinical samples has not significantly increased the diagnostic yield for melioidosis.

REFERENCES

1. Chakravorty A, et al. Melioidosis: An Updated Review. Aust J Gen Pract 2019; 48(5): 327–32.
2. Hotchkiss RS, et al. Sepsis and Septic Shock. Nat. Rev. Dis. Primers 2016; 2(1): 16045.
3. Lau SK, et al. Laboratory Diagnosis of Melioidosis: Past, Present and Future. Exp Biol Med (Maywood) 2015; 240(6): 742–51.
4. Sangwichian O, et al. Adapting Microarray Gene Expression Signatures for Early Melioidosis Diagnosis. J Clin Microbiol 2020; 58(7): e01906-19.
5. Standard operating procedure (SOP) for isolation of *Burkholderia pseudomallei* from clinical samples. Mahidol Oxford Tropical Medicine Research Unit(MORU). Version No: 1.5, MBL3-8–0M, November 2015.
6. Gassiep I, et al. Laboratory Safety: Handling *Burkholderia pseudomallei* Isolates Without a Biosafety Cabinet. J Clin Microbiol 2021; 59(7): e0042421.
7. Limmathurotsakul D, et al. Defining the True Sensitivity of Culture for the Diagnosis of Melioidosis Using Bayesian Latent Class Models. PLoS One 2010; 5(8): e12485.
8. Hoffmaster AR, et al. Melioidosis Diagnostic Workshop, 2013. Emerg Infect Dis 2015; 21(2): e141045.
9. Tellapragada C, et al. Improved Detection of *Burkholderia pseudomallei* from Non-Blood Clinical Specimens Using Enrichment Culture and PCR: Narrowing Diagnostic Gap in Resource-Constrained Settings. Trop Med Int Health 2017; 22(7): 866–70.
10. Dance DAB, et al. The Cost-Effectiveness of the Use of Selective Media for the Diagnosis of Melioidosis in Different Settings. PLoS Negl Trop Dis 2019; 13(7): e0007598.

11. Chantratita N, et al. Biological Relevance of Colony Morphology and Phenotypic Switching by *Burkholderia pseudomallei*. J Bacteriol 2007; 189(3): 807–17.
12. Hemarajata P, et al. *Burkholderia pseudomallei*: Challenges for the Clinical Microbiology Laboratory. J Clin Microbiol 2016; 54(12): 2866–73.
13. Trunck LA, et al. Molecular Basis of Rare Aminoglycoside Susceptibility and Pathogenesis of *Burkholderia pseudomallei* Clinical Isolates from Thailand. PLoS Negl Trop Dis 2009; 3(9): e519.
14. Podin Y, et al. *Burkholderia pseudomallei* isolates from Sarawak, Malaysian Borneo, are Predominantly Susceptible to Aminoglycosides and Macrolides. Antimicrob Agents Chemother 2014; 58(1): 162–6.
15. Lowe P, et al. Use of Various Common Isolation Media to Evaluate the New VITEK 2 Colorimetric GN Card for Identification of *Burkholderia pseudomallei*. J Clin Microbiol 2006; 44(3): 854–6.
16. Podin Y, et al. Reliability of Automated Biochemical Identification of *Burkholderia pseudomallei* Is Regionally Dependent. J Clin Microbiol 2013; 51(9): 3076–8.
17. Samosornsuk N, et al. Short Report: Evaluation of a Monoclonal Antibody-Based Latex Agglutination Test for Rapid Diagnosis of Septicemic Melioidosis. Am J Trop Med Hyg 1999; 61(5): 735–7.
18. Janesomboon S, et al. Detection and Differentiation of *Burkholderia* Species with Pathogenic Potential in Environmental Soil Samples. PLoS One 2021; 16(1): e0245175.
19. Naigowit P, et al. Application of Indirect Immunofluorescence Microscopy to Colony Identification of Pseudomonas Pseudomallei. Asian Pac J Allergy Immunol 1993; 11(2): 149–54.
20. Merritt A, et al. PCR-Based Identification of *Burkholderia pseudomallei*. Rev Inst Med Trop Sao Paulo 2006; 48(5): 239–44.
21. Rainbow L, et al. Distribution of Type III Secretion Gene Clusters in *Burkholderia pseudomallei, B. thailandensis and B. mallei*. J Med Microbiol 2002; 51(5): 374–84.
22. Lichtenegger S, et al. Development and Validation of a *Burkholderia pseudomallei* Core Genome Multilocus Sequence Typing Scheme to Facilitate Molecular Surveillance. J Clin Microbiol 2021; 59(8): e0009321.
23. Watthanaworawit W, et al. A Multi-Country Study Using MALDI-TOF Mass Spectrometry for Rapid Identification of *Burkholderia pseudomallei*. BMC Microbiol 2021; 21(1): 213.
24. Cheng AC, et al. Indirect Hemagglutination Assay in Patients with Melioidosis in Northern Australia. Am J Trop Med Hyg 2006; 74(2): 330–4.
25. Harris PN, et al. Clinical Features That Affect Indirect-Hemagglutination-Assay Responses to *Burkholderia pseudomallei*. Clin Vaccine Immunol 2009; 16(6): 924–30.
26. Corea E. Melioidosis: A Neglected Tropical Disease. Ceylon Med J 2018; 63(1): 1–4.
27. Fairley L, et al. Systematic Review and Meta-Analysis of Diagnostic Tests for Diagnosis of Melioidosis. Acta Trop 2021; 214: 105784.
28. Pumpuang A, et al. Comparison of O-Polysaccharide and Hemolysin Co-Regulated Protein as Target Antigens for Serodiagnosis of Melioidosis. PLoS Negl Trop Dis 2017; 11(3): e0005499.
29. Vadivelu J, et al. Diagnostic and Prognostic Value of an Immunofluorescent Assay for Melioidosis. Am J Trop Med Hyg 2000; 62(2): 297–300.
30. Phokrai P, et al. A Rapid Immunochromatography Test Based on Hcp1 Is a Potential Point-of-Care Test for Serological Diagnosis of Melioidosis. J Clin Microbiol 2018; 56(8): e00346-18.
31. Kohler C, et al. Rapid and Sensitive Multiplex Detection of *Burkholderia pseudomallei*-Specific Antibodies in Melioidosis Patients Based on a Protein Microarray Approach. PLoS Negl Trop Dis 2016; 10(7): e0004847.
32. Anuntagool N, et al. Monoclonal Antibody-Based Rapid Identification of *Burkholderia pseudomallei* in Blood Culture Fluid from Patients with Community-Acquired Septicemia. J Med Microbiol 2000; 49(12): 1075–78.

33. DeMers HL, et al. Detection and Quantification of the Capsular Polysaccharide of *Burkholderia pseudomallei* in Serum and Urine Samples from Melioidosis Patients. Microbiol Spectr 2022; 10 (4): e0076522.
34. Currie BJ, et al. What is The Role of Lateral Flow Immunoassay for the Diagnosis of Melioidosis? Open Forum Infect Dis 2022; 9(5): ofac149.
35. Radhakrishnan A, et al. Clinico-Microbiological Description and Evaluation of Rapid Lateral Flow Immunoassay and PCR for Detection of *Burkholderia pseudomallei* from Patients Hospitalized with Sepsis and Pneumonia: A Twenty-One Months Study from Odisha, India. Acta Trop 2021; 221: 105994.
36. Amornchai P, et al. Evaluation of Antigen-Detecting and Antibody-Detecting Diagnostic Test Combinations for Diagnosing Melioidosis. PLoS Negl Trop Dis 2021; 15(11): e0009840.
37. Amornchai P, et al. Sensitivity and Specificity of DPP® Fever Panel II Asia in the Diagnosis of Malaria, Dengue and Melioidosis. J Med Microbiol 2022; 71(8).
38. Gassiep I, et al. Diagnosis of Melioidosis: The Role of Molecular Techniques. Future Microbiol 2021; 16: 271–88.
39. Meumann EM, et al. Clinical Evaluation of a Type III Secretion System Real-Time PCR Assay for Diagnosing Melioidosis. J Clin Microbiol 2006; 44(8): 3028–30.
40. Gal D, et al. Short Report: Application of a Polymerase Chain Reaction to Detect *Burkholderia pseudomallei* in Clinical Specimens from Patients with Suspected Melioidosis. Am J Trop Med Hyg 2005; 73(6): 1162–4.
41. Chantratita N, et al. Loop-Mediated Isothermal Amplification Method Targeting The TTS1 Gene Cluster for Detection of *Burkholderia pseudomallei* and Diagnosis of Melioidosis. J Clin Microbiol 2008; 46(2): 568–73.
42. Peng Y, et al. Rapid Detection of *Burkholderia pseudomallei* With a Lateral Flow Recombinase Polymerase Amplification Assay. PLoS One 2019; 14(7): e0213416.
43. Saxena A, et al. Development of a Rapid and Sensitive Recombinase Polymerase Amplification-Lateral Flow Assay for Detection of *Burkholderia mallei*. Transbound Emerg Dis 2019; 66(2): 1016–22.
44. Schully KL, et al. Next-Generation Diagnostics for Melioidosis: Evaluation of a Prototype i-STAT Cartridge to Detect *Burkholderia pseudomallei* Biomarkers. Clin Infect Dis 2019; 69(3): 421–27.
45. CLSI. Methods for antimicrobial dilution and disk susceptibility testing of infrequently isolated or fastidious bacteria. 3rd ed. CLSI guideline M45. Wayne, PA: Clinical and Laboratory Standards Institute; 2015.
46. British Society for Antimicrobial Chemotherapy. Standing committee on susceptibility testing version 13.0, 10-06–2014. The global health network. Centre for tropical medicine and global health. UK: University of Oxford; 2014.
47. Dance DAB, et al. Interpreting Burkholderia *pseudomallei* Disc Diffusion Susceptibility Test Results by the EUCAST Method. Clin Microbiol Infect 2021; 27(6): 827–29.
48. Wuthiekanun V, et al. Trimethoprim/sulfamethoxazole Resistance in Clinical Isolates of Burkholderia *pseudomallei*. J Antimicrob Chemother 2005; 55(6): 1029–31.

Melioidosis

Pulmonary and Other Systemic Manifestations

Prasanta R Mohapatra

Department of Pulmonary Medicine and Critical Care,
All India Institute of Medical Sciences, Bhubaneswar, India

Contents

DOI: 10.1201/9781003324010-6

INTRODUCTION

Melioidosis is a disease caused by an environmental Gram-negative bacillus called *Burkholderia pseudomallei*. This disease typically manifests with acute melioidosis as pneumonia, sepsis, and multi-organ abscesses (Figure 6.1), with a variable high mortality rate.

    Burkholderia pseudomallei infections usually present as acute cases; about 15% of cases present as chronic or, uncommonly, can be latent with dormant bacilli. This disease frequently presents as a sub-clinical disease in immunocompetent individuals who cleared the infection due to immunity.

CLINICAL FEATURES

Melioidosis is a tropical infectious disease with various clinical presentations (Figure 6.1), and its severity varies from a fulminant septic illness to a slow-growing chronic infection. The clinical presentation of melioidosis depends on the site of the spread of the infection, bacterial load, virulence, and host immunity. Clinically, cases often have a non-specific presentation and may present from an acute fulminant condition to a very sluggish course of disease with a varied period of asymptomatic diseases. The presence of broad-based signs and symptoms can overlap with other diseases, resembling other conditions and often delaying melioidosis diagnosis and management (Table 6.1). Melioidosis is nicknamed 'the great mimicker.' Melioidosis is grossly underdiagnosed across the tropics, probably due to a lack of awareness and multiple symptoms that imitate other diseases without specific identifying features.

WHEN TO SUSPECT ACUTE MELIOIDOSIS

- A patient from an endemic area, exposures to dust, barefoot exposures to soil, mud, or water (contaminated environment)
- A patient with diabetes mellitus
- A patient with an acute/prolonged high-grade fever, not suggestive of any other cause
- Progressive pneumonia (chest radiograph deteriorating within a few days) not responding to commonly used antibiotics
- Visceral involvement like liver and/or spleen suggests multiple abscesses. An abdominal ultrasound/CT scan should be done to confirm or exclude other visceral abscesses

ACUTE MELIOIDOSIS

The most common type is acute melioidosis, defined as less than 2 months of symptoms. Patients with an acute infection account for nearly 85% of cases.[1] The incubation period

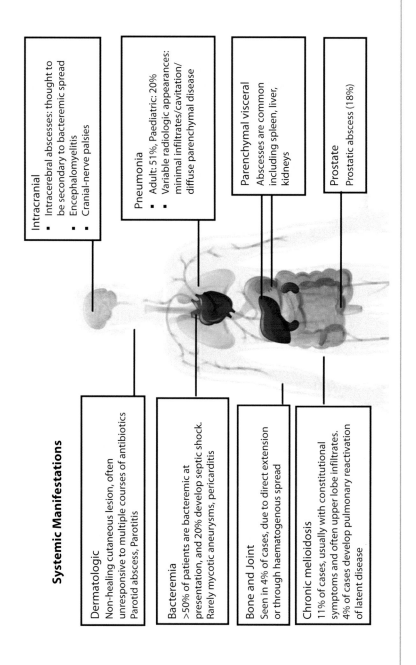

Systemic Manifestations

Intracranial
- Intracerebral abscesses: thought to be secondary to bacteremic spread
- Encephalomyelitis
- Cranial-nerve palsies

Pneumonia
- Adult: 51%, Paediatric: 20%
- Variable radiologic appearances: minimal infiltrates/cavitation/diffuse parenchymal disease

Parenchymal visceral
Abscesses are common including spleen, liver, kidneys

Prostate
Prostatic abscess (18%)

Dermatologic
Non-healing cutaneous lesion, often unresponsive to multiple courses of antibiotics
Parotid abscess, Parotitis

Bacteremia
>50% of patients are bacteremic at presentation, and 20% develop septic shock. Rarely mycotic aneurysms, pericarditis

Bone and Joint
Seen in 4% of cases, due to direct extension or through haematogenous spread

Chronic melioidosis
11% of cases, usually with constitutional symptoms and often upper lobe infiltrates. 4% of cases develop pulmonary reactivation of latent disease

FIGURE 6.1 Range of clinical manifestations after infection with *B. pseudomallei.*

TABLE 6.1 Comparison of clinical presentations worldwide

CLINICAL PRESENTATION	ODISHA[30]	INDIA[31,32]	AUSTRALIA[1,7,33]	MALAYSIA[34,35]	SINGAPORE[36,37]	THAILAND[14,38-40]
Fever	40/47 (85)	21/32 (79)	—		293/372 (79)	95/134 (71)
Pulmonary Infection	7/47 (14.8)	53/226 (23)	412/763 (54)	119/128 (93)	203/614 (33)	121/247 (49)
Skin/Soft Tissue Involvement	6 (12.7)	23/180 (13)	123/761 (16)	225/537 (42)	65/372 (17)	35/247 (14)
Bone and Joint Infection	2 (4.2)	36/226 (16)	22/597 (4)	99/402 (25)	2/372 (1)	35/247 (14)
Genitourinary Infection	1 (2.1)	5/180 (3)	—	35/402 (9)		8/134 (6)
Neurological Infection	5 (10.6)	19/180 (11)	22/751 (4)	21/370 (6)	2/372 (1)	2/30 (7)
Liver Abscess	2 (7.6)	20/180 (11)	17/597 (3)	46/537 (9)		93/247 (14)
Splenic Abscess	2 (7.6)	20/226 (9)	30/597 (5)	45/537 (8)		68/247 (14)
Prostate Abscess	2	8/226 (4)	83/408 (20)	5/225 (2)		13/155 (8)
Parotid Abscess	3 (14)	7/226 (3)	2/794 (.2)			5/134 (4)
Pericardial Effusion/Involvement	1 (2.1)	3/180 (2)	4/540 (1)	1/67 (1)	2/372 (1)	
Septic Shock	5 (10.6)	32/180 (18)	174/715 (24)	93/225 (41)		26/134 (19)
Bacteremia	5 (10.6)	87/226(38)	477/794 (60)	391/537 (73)	592/986 (60)	491/847 (56)
Mortality	7 (14.8)	32/180 (18)	118/794 (15)	212/527 (40)	260/614 (42)	1205/2913 (41)

Note: (—) no data

of melioidosis is 9 days (range from 1 to 21 days).[2] There may be a site of injection of *B. pseudomallei* in the mucosal surface or damaged skin. Careful history taking and examination may give a clue for cutaneous entry. After mucosal entry, it disseminates to various cells of the body.[3]

CHRONIC MELIOIDOSIS

Chronic melioidosis is defined as an illness of melioidosis for more than 2 months.[4] Chronic melioidosis occurred in nearly 11% of patients infected with *B. pseudomallei*.[1] Prolonged fever of unknown origin may be a typical presentation of chronic melioidosis, and at times it mimics tuberculosis. The persistent symptoms for more than 2 months accounted for nearly 10% of all cases. In a study over 20 years on 540 patients in Australia, the main presenting clinical feature was pneumonia (over half of the patients), followed by genito-urinary infection (14%), dermatologic infection mostly slow course (13%), bacteremia without definite evident focus (11%), septic arthritis or osteomyelitis (4%), and neurologic involvement (3%).[1] About 4% of patients had no evident focus of infection. Over half of the patients had bacteremia at presentation, and septic shock developed in approximately one-fifth of patients.[1]

PNEUMONIA

Pneumonia is the most common presentation in over half of the cases. Additionally, 20% of melioidosis patients develop secondary pneumonia along with other manifestations.[5] Bacteremia is commonly detected in patients with pneumonia and has been demonstrated in more than 60% of patients. Pneumonic melioidosis patients present with dyspnea and a productive cough.[6] Patient presentation may start with pneumonia or symptoms of any other system involvement. Respiratory disease is usually an early presentation, followed by bacteremic spread to different organs and viscera like the prostate, spleen, liver, and, occasionally, the central nervous system (CNS).[1] A bacteremic patient usually presents with systemic symptoms such as a high-grade fever. Other symptoms related to localized organ involvement may rapidly make the condition worse. Some patients may develop sepsis. Septic shock due to melioidosis accounts for 21–34% of patients.[1,7] It may be associated with the involvement of other systems like the spleen, kidney, and prostatic abscesses. Pneumonia can be atypical and may be associated with pleural effusion. This multi-systemic involvement is primarily due to hematogenous spread.[6] Serial chest radiograph may show a rapid progression; it may start with lung infiltrates, which used to coalesce, develop focal to diffuse consolidation, central caseation, and necrosis, which lead to a breakdown, cavitation, and abscess formation, with or without fluid level.[8] If it remains untreated or wrongly treated, other organs get involved due to disseminated infections through the bloodstream. Internal organ, intra-abdominal abscesses, along with foci in the lungs, are also common. Geographical variations in the manifestations like suppurative parotitis, which were

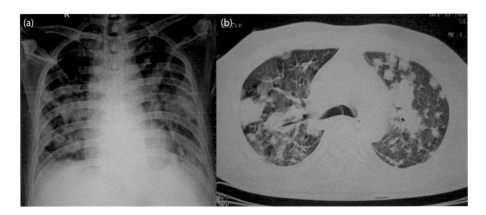

FIGURE 6.2   Chest X-ray (A) in the posteroanterior view of a 40-year-old man showing bilateral consolidation and multiple non-homogenous opacity. Chest computed tomography (B) in the transverse plane of same patient showing a cotton-ball like lesion in the background of bilateral consolidation and multiple dense cotton-ball like opacity.

observed in up to 40% of cases, are mainly seen in children in countries like Thailand, Laos, and Cambodia.[9]

The radiographic presentations of melioidosis, such as the acute onset of pneumonia with lobar patch patchy alveolar infiltrate with or without a cavity, bilateral diffuse patchy alveolar infiltration, or multiple nodular lesions (Figures 6.2 and 6.3) and may have a predilection for upper-lobe like lesion of tuberculosis. But the rapid progression of patchy alveolar infiltrates with early cavitation can be multiple, and bigger sizes are common. Unlike lobar pneumonia, multiple-lobe involvement can be seen in about 30% of patients.[5] Pleural effusion can be a chronic presentation, and empyema

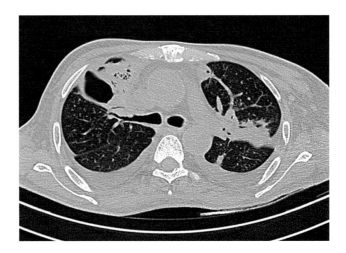

FIGURE 6.3   Computed tomography of the thorax showing bilateral consolidation and pleural effusion with a thick-walled abscess in the right upper lobe.

along with lung abscess are common in both acute and chronic cases.[10] Hilar and mediastinal lymphadenopathy are also increasingly being detected with the availability of computed tomography (CT) scans. Ultrasound and CT scans may reveal many concomitant silent abscesses in the neck and abdominal organs like the spleen, liver, prostate, or abdominal lymph nodes. CT thorax is more valuable in finding small consolidations or abscesses, even with a normal chest radiograph. Hemoptysis can be a presentation in melioidosis.[11] *B. pseudomallei* rarely presents as hospital-acquired pneumonia.[12] Common differential diagnoses of pulmonary melioidosis[12] are bronchogenic carcinoma,[12] staphylococcal pneumonia, and tuberculosis.

PULMONARY MELIOIDOSIS IN CYSTIC FIBROSIS

Cystic fibrosis (CF) is mostly a disease in the northern hemisphere and Western countries. Many cases of melioidosis have been reported without travel history in CF patients. Incidental isolation of *B. pseudomallei* was observed in 42% of patients with increased sputum production and cough.[13] Refractory bronchopulmonary sepsis can be a clinical presentation.[13] Other *Burkholderia* spp. (e.g., *B. cepacia,* etc.) are relatively common in CF patients and are also likely to be misidentified. A high index of suspicion for the diagnosis of the *Burkholderia* group is important.[13]

SEPTICEMIA

Sepsis is a serious presentation of melioidosis. There is evidence of primary localized infection and disease spreading through different routes. From the local focus of infection, metastatic spread of infection is common during bacteremia, mainly seen in the lungs. Multi-focal pneumonia may get organized or spread to the liver, spleen, kidneys, prostate (multiple abscesses), skin and soft tissues (cellulitis, pustules), bones, and joints, although any site may be vulnerable.

PYREXIA OF UNKNOWN ORIGIN

Melioidosis can be a cause of fever of unknown origin. The fever is usually prolonged and may be high-grade with fluctuation. Bacteraemia may be associated intermittently and deep-seated multiple visceral abscesses. It should be diligently sought.

PROSTATIC MELIOIDOSIS

Melioidosis involves the prostate in about 20% of male patients. These prostatic abscesses are less commonly detected (1–13%) in places like Southeast Asia, possibly due to decreased clinical and radiographic detection for various reasons.[14] Prostatic involvement or prostatic abscess usually presents urinary symptoms like painful or difficult urination with increased frequency and urgency, which may be associated with retention or incontinence.[15,16] Leukocyturia is the most reliable finding. All prostatic abscesses due to melioidosis had urinary leukocyte counts of at least $50 \times 10^6/L$.[16] The value is correlated with a 100% negative predictive value. A transrectal ultrasound (TRUS) and CT scan evaluation are helpful imaging modalities. Commonly, the abscesses are large (>4.5 cm) and may involve both lobes or multi-loculated.[15,17] For diagnosing prostatic abscesses in melioidosis, ultrasonography has a sensitivity of 85%, compared with 99% by CT.[18] An aspirated or pus drained from the abscess is the most important specimen for bacterial culture.[19,20] A microbiological culture of the abscess fluid was used to confirm *B. pseudomallei*. Blood specimens in some patients also yield the diagnosis due to dissemination into the bloodstream. The same can also be isolated from urine.[19] Smaller abscesses (<1 cm) (Figure 6.4E) are usually better managed with antimicrobial therapy, whereas a larger abscess needs prompt drainage.[15,16,19] The relapse can occur in prostatic melioidosis. Culture-confirmed relapses have been reported in about 11–12% of patients after being discharged from their initial hospitalization.[21]

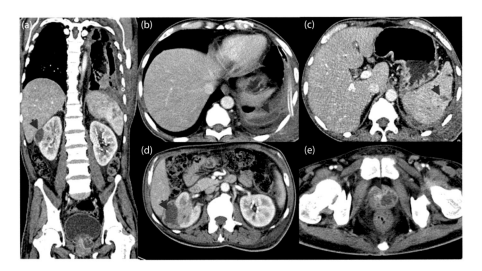

FIGURE 6.4 Computed tomography in the coronal plane (A) showing renal abscess and empyema with pleural thickening. Transverse plane (B to E) of the same patient showing empyema (B), splenic abscess (C), renal abscess (D) and prostatic abscess (E).

CUTANEOUS MELIOIDOSIS

Cutaneous melioidosis is infrequently seen, contrary to systemic melioidosis. It should be suspected in travelers who are residing or returning from endemic countries. It usually presents with cutaneous abscesses, cellulitis, or ulcerations. Surgery may be needed in some patients and warrants follow-up for at least 1 year.[22] Cutaneous melioidosis seems to be expected in relation to contaminated items used as cleaning materials.[23,24]

NEUROLOGIC MELIOIDOSIS

Neurologic melioidosis usually manifests as brainstem encephalitis, frequently with cranial-nerve palsies (seventh cranial nerve involvement is common), or as myelitis with peripheral motor weakness.[1] Encephalomyelitis and brain abscess are the two most common types of disease. Encephalomyelitis in adults (39%) and brain abscess in children (44%) are commonly observed. Fever, headache, altered consciousness, neck stiffness, seizures, unilateral weakness, paraplegia, quadriplegia, and cranial nerve palsies are also common. Facial nerve involvement is common among other cranial nerves. More than 50% of cases have pulmonary involvement.[25] Diagnosis of neuro-melioidosis remains challenging.

WARNING SIGN OF MELIOIDOSIS

- Acute high-grade fever
- Difficulty in breathing
- Symptoms of pneumonia such as fever, respiratory distress, cough
- Shock (hypotension)
- Systemic symptoms (nausea, poor appetite, lethargy)

SEPTIC ARTHRITIS AND OSTEOMYELITIS

Septic arthritis and osteomyelitis are uncommonly due to *B. pseudomallei*. But again, it is usually seen in endemic areas. In one study cohort, 25.4% had primary septic arthritis, and 31.7% had primary osteomyelitis. Septic arthritis of the lower limb was associated with a 27.5% risk of osteomyelitis of adjacent bones.[26] About 48% of all cases of bacterial-culture-proven septic arthritis were due to *B. pseudomallei*, and 8.4% of patients had bone or joint involvement in a study in Thailand.[27,28]

The delay in the diagnosis and inappropriate antibiotic treatment worsens the condition. The broad-spectrum empirical antibiotics are usually inadequate in controlling *B. pseudomallei*. The guidelines for using empirical antibiotics for community-acquired pneumonia, particularly in endemic regions, should include the antibiotics against *B. pseudomallei* in patients with associated risk factors for melioidosis. However, the laboratory needs to maximize the culture results and identify *B. pseudomallei*. But in routine practice, a delay in confirming the identification of *B. pseudomallei* is plausible, mainly when laboratories are unfamiliar with this organism.[29] When empirical treatment has already started, it may be challenging to isolate *B. pseudomallei* by cultures. Therefore, obtaining blood and other tissue fluid specimens is essential before therapy.

DIAGNOSIS

The culture of the organism from any patient sample remains the criterion for the diagnosis of melioidosis. The specimens can be blood, aspirated pus, respiratory secretions, debrided tissue, urine, cerebrospinal fluid (CSF), and swabs from soft tissue lesions. Bacteremia was found in 38–73% of cases.[14] Clinical suspicion is the essential step in the diagnosis. Patients with uncontrolled diabetes, typical history of exposure in a known endemic area around the rainy season, and suggestive clinical features (like fever, pneumonia, multiple or single abscesses, especially in the different soft-tissue organs) should be suspected case of melioidosis (Figure 6.5) and should be treated empirically. However, based on the clinical course and presentation, patients without risk factors should undergo laboratory testing to confirm or alternate diagnosis of melioidosis.[41] The laboratory diagnosis details are available in Chapter 5 of this book.

Clinical Clues

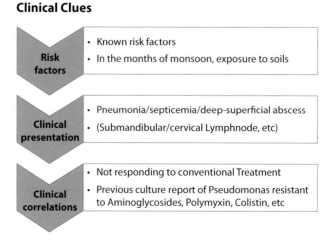

Risk factors
- Known risk factors
- In the months of monsoon, exposure to soils

Clinical presentation
- Pneumonia/septicemia/deep-superficial abscess
- (Submandibular/cervical Lymphnode, etc)

Clinical correlations
- Not responding to conventional Treatment
- Previous culture report of Pseudomonas resistant to Aminoglycosides, Polymyxin, Colistin, etc

FIGURE 6.5 Clinical clues to suspect melioidosis.

MICROBIOLOGICAL DIAGNOSIS

LABORATORY INVESTIGATION FOR MELIOIDOSIS

- Routine tests: Complete blood count, renal and liver functions, blood sugar
- Blood cultures (from two different sites at the same time before the antibiotic started)
- Cultures from the abscess, joint aspirate, CSF, sputum, or throat swab as indicated
- Urine culture and microscopic examination of urine

Culture: Overall, the sensitivity of blood culture is about 60%. The culture of the soft tissue fluid, throat, or rectal swabs can be used.[42,43] Urine is also suggested in all cases of suspected melioidosis, and centrifuged deposits are preferred.[44] Abscess fluid collected from different organs, soft-tissue abscess, pus, and pleural fluid is also ideal for culture.

The Active Melioidosis Detect (AMD)™ lateral flow immunoassay (LFI), (InBios International, United States) a lateral flow assay (LFA) detecting *B. pseudomallei* capsular polysaccharide (CPS) via a monoclonal antibody is becoming popular as a point-of-care (POC) test.

IMAGING

Various imaging modalities are available to support the diagnosis of melioidosis. The lung is commonly involved. Common chest radiographic features are multi-focal nodular and patchy consolidation with cavitary lesions (figures 6.2, 6.3 and 6.4).[8] Chest radiographs may also have rapidly involved patchy consolidation and enlarging coalescent nodules, succeeding breakdown, and thick-walled cavitation.[8] The lung consolidation can be in any lobe of the lung and, gradually progress to abscesses, and abscesses break down to cavity formation.[8] Sub-acute and chronic pulmonary infections may present with slowly progressive upper-lobe consolidation with pleomorphic features that mimic tuberculosis.[8,45] Pleural effusion and empyema are commonly seen with sub-pleural involvement and rupture of a sub-pleural abscess to pleural spaces. In chronic pulmonary melioidosis, the resolution is unlikely to heal with scarring and calcification.[8,46] Hilar lymphadenopathy is relatively uncommon in melioidosis and is more likely to represent tuberculosis in regions of endemicity.[8,45,47] CT scans of the thorax may give better clues than chest radiographs. The consolidation, abscess formation, and early cavitation are better appreciated in CT Thorax.[8]

Ultrasound is beneficial in detecting superficial and deep visceral abscesses in diagnosing melioidosis.[48] Liver and spleen abscesses are appreciated as small target-like hypoechoic lesions and clinically correlated with melioidosis.[47,48] In the CT scan, the liver abscesses may occasionally show honeycomb signs due to multiple small similar-sized locations separated by thin septa. For visceral abscesses, CT scans seem to be better than ultrasonography.[49]

Magnetic resonance imaging (MRI) has been demonstrated as a better diagnostic aid and is seen as either ring-enhancing lesions or enhancement leptomeninges.[50] MRI has been more sensitive for diagnosing CNS melioidosis, particularly in detecting cerebral edema and micro-abscesses.[47]

DIFFERENTIAL DIAGNOSIS OF PULMONARY MANIFESTATIONS[12]

Acute Severe Cases

- Pneumonia
- Community-acquired septicaemia
- Lung abscesses, particularly *Staphylococcus aureus*
- Tuberculosis

Disseminated/Chronic Pulmonary Tuberculosis

- Septic pulmonary embolism
- Multi-organ abscess, with subcutaneous lesion

MANAGEMENT

Early diagnosis and the early administration of appropriate antibiotics are crucial for managing melioidosis. In addition to appropriate antimicrobial therapy, any localized collection or abscesses needs drainage, and infected superficial tissue needs debridement.

GENERAL TREATMENT FOR MELIOIDOSIS

- Correction of fluids, electrolytes, and acid-base imbalance
- Insulin therapy for diabetic patients
- Incision and drainage of the abscess. Patients with liver abscesses larger than 5 cm × 5 cm should be referred to an interventional radiologist or surgeon for drainage by pigtail catheter or other modalities.
- Pulse oximetry or arterial blood gas-monitoring in severely ill cases when patients may require respiratory support
- Standard precaution procedures for infection control should be implemented in the care of these patients

The antibiotic management of melioidosis comprises an early intensive therapy of an intravenous antibiotic such as ceftazidime, meropenem, or imipenem for 2–4 weeks; trimethoprim-sulfamethoxazole remained the preferred agent for eradication therapy as per the 2020 revised Darwin melioidosis treatment guideline.[51] The management is discussed in a separate chapter 9 under Drug Management in this book.

If untreated, the overall mortality of bacteremic melioidosis may reach up to 100%, but early and appropriate management can reduce the mortality to a very minimal level. The involvement of the lung carries a mortality rate of over 50%.

LONG-TERM FOLLOW UP

FOLLOW UP AFTER ERADICATION PHASE

At least for 5 years (majority of patients have diabetes, and they will be followed for the life for their diabetes)

- Interval of follow-up: every 6 months, or as needed depending on severity
- Look for evidence of relapses, e.g., prolonged fever, acute pneumonia, musculoskeletal abscesses, liver, and splenic abscesses

REFERENCES

1. Currie BJ, et al. The Epidemiology and Clinical Spectrum of Melioidosis: 540 Cases from the 20 Year Darwin Prospective Study. PLoS Negl Trop Dis 2010; 4(11): e900.
2. Currie BJ, et al. Melioidosis: Acute and Chronic Disease, Relapse and Re-Activation. Trans R Soc Trop Med Hyg 2000; 94(3): 301–4.
3. Wiersinga WJ, et al. Melioidosis. Nat Rev Dis Primers 2018; 4: 17107.
4. Currie BJ, et al. Endemic Melioidosis in Tropical Northern Australia: A 10-Year Prospective Study and Review of the Literature. Clin Infect Dis 2000; 31(4): 981–6.
5. Meumann EM, et al. Clinical Features and Epidemiology of Melioidosis Pneumonia: Results from a 21-Year Study and Review of the Literature. Clin Infect Dis 2012; 54(3): 362–9.
6. Currie BJ. Melioidosis: Evolving Concepts in Epidemiology, Pathogenesis, and Treatment. Semin Respir Crit Care Med 2015; 36(1): 111–25.
7. Stewart JD, et al. The Epidemiology and Clinical Features of Melioidosis in Far North Queensland: Implications for Patient Management. PLoS Negl Trop Dis 2017; 11(3): e0005411.
8. Burivong W, et al. Thoracic Radiologic Manifestations of Melioidosis. Curr Probl Diagn Radiol 2012; 41(6): 199–209.
9. Pagnarith Y, et al. Emergence of Pediatric Melioidosis in Siem Reap, Cambodia. Am J Trop Med Hyg 2010; 82(6): 1106–12.
10. Mohanty S, et al. A Case of Systemic Melioidosis: Unravelling the Etiology of Chronic Unexplained Fever with Multiple Presentations. Pneumonol Alergol Pol 2016; 84(2): 121–5.

11. Kwon EH, et al. Distinguishing Respiratory Features of Category A/B Potential Bioterrorism Agents from Community-Acquired Pneumonia. Health Secur 2018; 16(4): 224–38.

12. Virk HS, et al. Melioidosis: A Neglected Cause of Community-Acquired Pneumonia. Semin Respir Crit Care Med 2020; 41(4): 496–508.

13. Geake JB, et al. An International, Multicentre Evaluation and Description of *Burkholderia Pseudomallei* Infection in Cystic Fibrosis. BMC Pulm Med 2015; 15: 116.

14. Gassiep I, et al. Human Melioidosis. Clin Microbiol Rev 2020; 33(2): e00006–19. https://doi.org/10.1128/CMR.00006-19

15. Wahab AA, et al. A Fatal Case of Primary Melioidotic Prostatic Abscess: The Peril of Poor Drug Compliance. Trop Biomed 2020; 37(3): 560–65.

16. Kozlowska J, et al. Prostatic Abscess Due to *Burkholderia pseudomallei*: Facilitating Diagnosis to Optimize Management. Am J Trop Med Hyg 2018; 98(1): 227–30.

17. Chong Vh VH, et al. Urogenital Melioidosis: A Review of Clinical Presentations, Characteristic and Outcomes. Med J Malaysia 2014; 69(6): 257–60.

18. Morse LP, et al. Prostatic Abscess Due to *Burkholderia pseudomallei*: 81 Cases from a 19-Year Prospective Melioidosis Study. J Urol 2009; 182(2): 542–7; discussion 47.

19. Tan G, et al. Prostatic Melioidosis Rarely Reported in China: Two Cases Report and Literatures Review. Int J Clin Exp Med 2015; 8(11): 21830–2.

20. Chee YC, et al. An Unusual Case of Primary Melioidotic Prostatic Abscess Complicated by Perianal Abscess. IDCases 2018; 11: 51–52.

21. Chien JM, et al. Factors Affecting Clinical Outcomes in the Management of Melioidosis in Singapore: A 16-Year Case Series. BMC Infect Dis 2018; 18(1): 482.

22. Fertitta L, et al. Cutaneous Melioidosis: A Review of the Literature. Int J Dermatol 2019; 58(2): 221–7.

23. Gal D, et al. Contamination of Hand Wash Detergent Linked to Occupationally Acquired Melioidosis. Am J Trop Med Hyg 2004; 71(3): 360–2.

24. Clark B, et al. Clinical Features and Outcome of Patients with Cutaneous Melioidosis During a Nosocomial Outbreak in a Temperate Region of Australia. Intern Med J 2018; 48(4): 461–65.

25. Wongwandee M, et al. Central Nervous System Melioidosis: A Systematic Review of Individual Participant Data of Case Reports and Case Series. PLoS Negl Trop Dis 2019; 13(4): e0007320.

26. Shetty RP, et al. Management of Melioidosis Osteomyelitis and Septic Arthritis. Bone Joint J 2015; 97-b(2): 277–82.

27. Teparrukkul P, et al. Clinical Epidemiology of Septic Arthritis Caused by *Burkholderia pseudomallei* and Other Bacterial Pathogens in Northeast Thailand. Am J Trop Med Hyg 2017; 97(6): 1695–701.

28. Teparrakkul P, et al. Rheumatological Manifestations in Patients with Melioidosis. Southeast Asian J Trop Med Public Health 2008; 39(4): 649–55.

29. Peacock SJ, et al. Management of Accidental Laboratory Exposure to *Burkholderia pseudomallei* and *B. mallei*. Emerg Infect Dis 2008; 14(7): e2.

30. Behera B, et al. Melioidosis in Odisha: A Clinico-Microbiological and Epidemiological Description of Culture-Confirmed Cases Over a 2-Year Period. Indian J Med Microbiol 2019; 37(3): 430–32.

31. Gopalakrishnan R, et al. Melioidosis: An Emerging Infection in India. J Assoc Physicians India 2013; 61(9): 612–4.

32. Vidyalakshmi K, et al. Emerging Clinico-Epidemiological Trends in Melioidosis: Analysis of 95 Cases from Western Coastal India. Int J Infect Dis 2012; 16(7): e491–e7.

33. Malczewski AB, et al. Clinical Presentation of Melioidosis in Queensland, Australia. Trans R Soc Trop Med Hyg 2005; 99(11): 856–60.

34. Zueter A, et al. The Epidemiology and Clinical spectrum of Melioidosis in a Teaching Hospital in a North-Eastern State of Malaysia: A Fifteen-Year Review. BMC Infect Dis 2016; 16: 333.
35. How SH, et al. Melioidosis in Pahang, Malaysia. Med J Malaysia 2005; 60(5): 606–13.
36. Heng BH, et al. Epidemiological Surveillance of Melioidosis in Singapore. Ann Acad Med Singap 1998; 27(4): 478–84.
37. Pang L, et al. Melioidosis, Singapore, 2003-2014. Emerg Infect Dis 2018; 24(1): 140–3.
38. Limmathurotsakul D, et al. Increasing Incidence of Human Melioidosis in Northeast Thailand. Am J Trop Med Hyg 2010; 82(6): 1113–7.
39. Suputtamongkol Y, et al. Risk Factors for Melioidosis and Bacteremic Melioidosis. Clin Infect Dis 1999; 29(2): 408–13.
40. Churuangsuk C, et al. Characteristics, Clinical Outcomes and Factors Influencing Mortality of Patients with Melioidosis in Southern Thailand: A 10-Year Retrospective Study. Asian Pac J Trop Med 2016; 9(3): 256–60.
41. Hoffmaster AR, et al. Melioidosis Diagnostic Workshop, 2013. Emerg Infect Dis 2015; 21(2): e141045. https://doi.org/10.3201/eid2102.141045
42. Cheng AC, et al. Role of Selective and Nonselective Media for Isolation of *Burkholderia pseudomallei* from Throat Swabs of Patients with Melioidosis. J Clin Microbiol 2006; 44(6): 2316.
43. Wuthiekanun V, et al. Value of Throat Swab in Diagnosis of Melioidosis. J Clin Microbiol 2001; 39(10): 3801–2.
44. Limmathurotsakul D, et al. Role and Significance of Quantitative Urine Cultures in Diagnosis of Melioidosis. J Clin Microbiol 2005; 43(5): 2274–6.
45. Muttarak M, et al. Spectrum of Imaging Findings in Melioidosis. Br J Radiol 2009; 82(978): 514–21.
46. Reechaipichitkul W. Clinical Manifestation of Pulmonary Melioidosis in Adults. Southeast Asian J Trop Med Public Health 2004; 35(3): 664–9.
47. Lim KS, et al. Radiological Manifestations of Melioidosis. Clin Radiol 2010; 65(1): 66–72.
48. Wibulpolprasert B, et al. Visceral Organ Abscesses in Melioidosis: Sonographic Findings. J Clin Ultrasound 1999; 27(1): 29–34.
49. Khiangte HL, et al. A Retrospective Case-Control Study to Evaluate the Diagnostic Accuracy of Honeycomb Sign in Melioid Liver Abscess. Am J Trop Med Hyg 2018; 99(4): 852–57.
50. Currie BJ, et al. Neurological Melioidosis. Acta Trop 2000; 74(2–3): 145–51.
51. Sullivan RP, et al. 2020 Review and Revision of the 2015 Darwin Melioidosis Treatment Guideline; Paradigm Drift Not Shift. PLoS Negl Trop Dis 2020; 14(9): e0008659.

Radiological Imaging in Melioidosis

7

Suprava Naik

Department of Radiodiagnosis, All India Institute of Medical Sciences, Bhubaneswar, India

Ranjan Kumar Patel

Department of Radiodiagnosis, All India Institute of Medical Sciences, Bhubaneswar, India

Contents

INTRODUCTION

Melioidosis caused by Gram-negative aerobic bacteria *Burkholderia pseudomallei* is endemic in Southeast Asia, northern Australia, and many tropical countries. The bacteria reside in the soil and water of the endemic region and enter the human body through

DOI: 10.1201/9781003324010-7

skin abrasion, ingestion, or inhalation. Thus, an increased incidence may be anticipated in the endemic zone after rainfall and following natural disasters, such as tsunamis and cyclones.[1-4]

While melioidosis is more frequent in patients with underlying co-morbidities, such as diabetes mellitus, chronic kidney disease, alcoholism, underlying malignancy/haematological disorders, and immunosuppression, occupational exposure to soil is an important risk factor in patients without any underlying disease. The disseminated form is more frequent in diabetic patients. Of note, melioidosis is not common in patients with acquired immunodeficiency syndrome (AIDS).[1-4]

Clinical features are non-specific and can simulate other infections. Clinical presentation may vary from localized cutaneous infections at the inoculation site and chronic multi-system involvement simulating tuberculosis (TB) to acute fulminant sepsis and death. The acute septicaemic form carries very high mortality (>80%) unless treated in a timely manner with appropriate therapy.

The gold standard for diagnosis of melioidosis is the culture and isolation of *B. pseudomallei* from samples obtained from the patient. Treatment is also based upon definitive isolation of the organism on culture. Isolation of organisms in culture media may take days to weeks. So, imaging plays a vital role in the early identification of the site and extent of infection.

IMAGING

Melioidosis can involve every organ system of our body. The imaging findings are non-specific and mimic other bacterial infections. However, some imaging findings help raise the possibility of melioidosis in patients with proper clinical backgrounds. X-ray, computed tomography scan (CT scan), ultrasonography (USG), and magnetic resonance imaging (MRI) are very useful in confirming sites of infection. X-ray is useful in pulmonary and musculoskeletal involvement, USG in abdominal visceral and superficial soft-tissue involvement, CT scan in thoracic, abdominal, and visceral involvement, MRI in central nervous system (CNS) involvement and early bone changes that may not be evident on X-ray and CT scans.

It is also important in view of image-guided aspiration of small abscess from which the organism may be isolated by culture to increase diagnostic yield. Therapeutic image-guided drainage can be used as supportive therapy in case of a larger abscess. Imaging also helps assess the response to treatment and follow-up of patients on prolonged treatment.

THORACIC MANIFESTATIONS

The lung is the most common organ involved in melioidosis in approximately half of the patients. Respiratory system involvement in melioidosis is associated with unfavourable outcomes. The spectrum of imaging findings includes small nodules, consolidation, cavitations, and lung abscesses. These findings can be better visualized on CT scans (Figure 7.1).

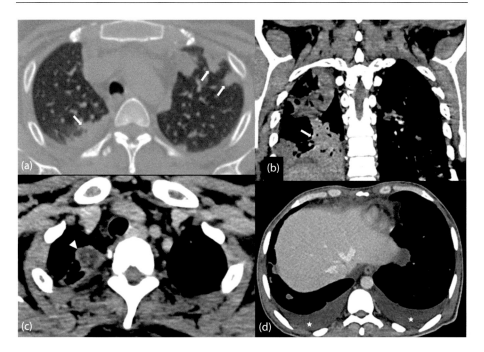

FIGURE 7.1 CT scan of the thorax in a 30-year-old male patient. The axial CT scan lung window (a), the coronal reformatted image of a mediastinal window (b), and axial mediastinal window (c) show areas of consolidation (arrows in a and b) in both lungs and abscess formation (arrowhead in c) in the right upper lobe. An axial contrast-enhanced CT scan in another patient (d) shows a small abscess in the right lower lobe and bilateral pleural effusion (asterisk).

Pulmonary melioidosis and pulmonary TB have many clinically and radiologically overlapping features. So, it is important to keep both differentials in mind, particularly in places where both are endemic. Consolidation in melioidosis commonly involves the upper lobe; however, the lung apex is relatively spared, unlike TB. Consolidations can progress rapidly, and thin-walled cavitation is common in melioidosis. Air-fluid levels within the cavities are unusual findings compared to TB and staphylococcal infection.[5,6] In disseminated infection, imaging looks like miliary TB. In the chronic stage of melioidosis, consolidations and cavitations are associated with surrounding fibrosis. Other thoracic findings include pleural effusion and empyema (Figure 7.1). Of note, intrathoracic lymphadenopathy is less common in melioidosis than TB.

ABDOMINOPELVIC MANIFESTATIONS

The spleen is the most common abdominal organ involved in melioidosis, followed by the liver. The kidney, prostate, and pancreas are relatively uncommon sites of involvement. The most common imaging findings are liver and splenic abscesses. Imaging

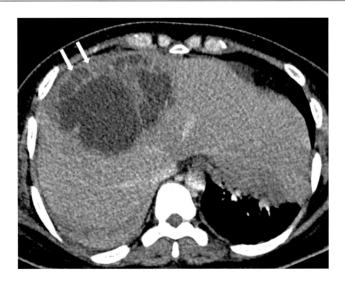

FIGURE 7.2   Contrast-enhanced CT scan of the abdomen in a 28-year-old female patient with melioidosis shows a liver abscess with internal septations. Peripherally arranged septation is giving a 'string of pearls' appearance (arrows).

shows single or multiple small discrete lesions and single or multiple multi-loculated lesions better visualized on USG and CT scans. Multiple septate micro-abscesses have been described as 'honeycomb' or 'string-of-pearls' signs, particularly in hepatic abscesses[6-8] (Figures 7.2 and 7.3). Abscesses may also show target appearance on USG (Figure 7.4). Subcapsular abscesses, when ruptured, lead to a localized intraperitoneal collection. Isolated splenic abscesses or combined splenic and liver abscesses raise suspicion of melioidosis, especially in patients with other co-morbidities or in patients living in the endemic zone who present with fever of unknown origin and/or abdominal pain.

Pancreatic involvement is seen as focal pancreatitis, a pancreatic abscess that may be multi-focal micro-abscesses to large focal abscesses. Peri-pancreatic inflammation, fat stranding, and splenic vein thrombosis may be associated. All these findings can be better appreciated in a contrast-enhanced CT scan of the abdomen. Pancreatic involvement is usually secondary to septicaemia; however, it can be due to contiguous spread.[9]

Genitourinary involvement is usually seen in the setting of chronic disease as a part of a disseminated form of melioidosis. Patients present with fever, dysuria, frequency, and flank pain. The prostate is the most common organ involved in the genitourinary system, followed by the kidney, urinary bladder, and seminal vesicle. Prostatic involvement is in the form of prostatic abscess or prostatitis, and renal involvement is in the form of pyelonephritis or renal abscesses. Renal, prostatic, and seminal vesicle abscesses may also show a multi-septated or honeycomb appearance. These are indistinguishable from other infective causes on imaging; however, simultaneous splenic or lung involvement in a proper clinical setting gives a clue to the diagnosis of melioidosis.[10]

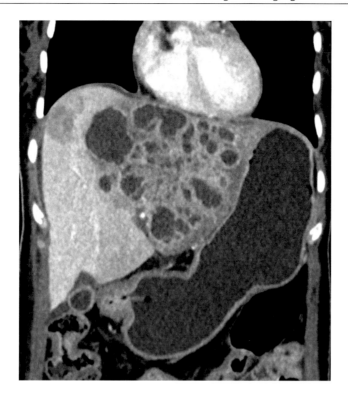

FIGURE 7.3 Coronal reformatted image of a contrast-enhanced CT scan of the abdomen of a melioidosis patient shows a large liver abscess with peripheral enhancement and enhancing internal septations having a 'honeycomb' appearance.

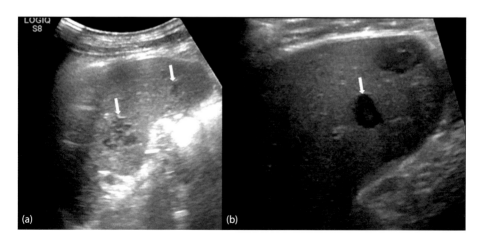

FIGURE 7.4 Abdominal ultrasonography (USG) in a melioidosis patient (a) shows multiple splenic abscesses (arrows). USG with a high-frequency transducer (b) shows 'target appearance' of the abscess (arrow in b).

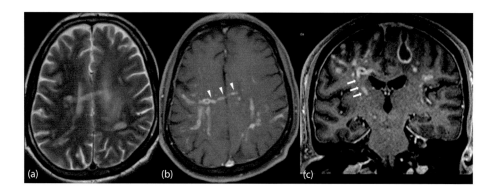

FIGURE 7.5   Axial T2W MRI (a) in a melioidosis patient shows multiple hyperintense lesions involving the white matter of the bilateral cerebral hemisphere and corpus callosum. Post-contrast axial (b) and coronal (c) T1WI show multiple small enhancing micro-abscesses extending along the white matter tracts: Corpus callosum (arrowheads in B) and corticospinal tract (arrows in c). One larger abscess in the left parietal lobe showed peripheral enhancement (c).

CNS INVOLVEMENT

CNS involvement occurs either as a part of the disseminated form or from contiguous spread from skull base osteomyelitis. CNS manifestations are meningitis, subdural empyema, encephalitis, cerebritis, and brain abscess. Brain abscesses in melioidosis are typically smaller in size, also termed micro-abscesses, extend along the white matter tracts, and commonly involve the brainstem and trigeminal nucleus (Figure 7.5). Contrast-enhanced MRI is the diagnostic modality of choice for the diagnosis of cerebritis, encephalitis, and meningitis. Brain abscesses can be seen as ring-enhancing lesions on post-contrast T1WI, and diffusion-weighted imaging (DWI) shows the central area of diffusion restriction. Due to the higher soft-tissue resolution of MRI, it can detect early changes in the brain and spine that may be missed by a CT scan.[11,12]

MUSCULOSKELETAL AND SOFT TISSUE INVOLVEMENT

Musculoskeletal involvement is often seen in the disseminated form of melioidosis, usually as a chronic and relapsing infection. Imaging shows features of osteomyelitis and septic arthritis with or without contiguous soft-tissue involvement in the form of pyomyositis and soft-tissue abscesses or cellulitis. An X-ray may show a permeative lesion in the involved bone. USG can demonstrate synovial effusion, peri-articular or soft-tissue

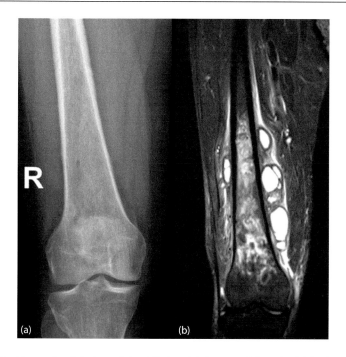

FIGURE 7.6 X-ray of a right knee joint AP view (a) shows mild cortical thinning and irregularity of the inner cortex involving the right lower femoral metaphyseal region. Coronal proton density fat suppression MRI of the lower femur of the patient (b) shows heterogeneously increased signal intensity in the metaphysis and adjacent diaphysis of the right femur. Multiple small abscesses with internal septations are seen in adjacent muscles.

abscess, and guide for aspiration. MRI can show early bone changes that can be missed by X-ray or a CT scan. MRI shows synovial enhancement in post-contrast T1WI, marrow oedema in the form of altered signal intensity in the bone in T1 and T2WI, and intraosseous abscess. It can also better visualize soft-tissue abscesses that can be unilocular or septated (Figure 7.6). Weight-bearing joints like knee, ankle, and hip joints are commonly involved. In one of the largest series of melioidosis, the femur and knee joint was the most common site of involvement.[6,13,14] Spinal melioidosis mimics tubercular spondylitis. Psoas abscess has also been reported in melioidosis. Disseminated infection may lead to cellulitis and soft-tissue abscesses as well. *B. pseudomallei* can cause localized intramuscular infection without associated bone or joint disease.

OTHER ORGAN INVOLVEMENT

Any organ can be affected by melioidosis. Abscesses may occur in the skin, subcutaneous tissues, and lymph nodes. Rare sites of involvement include parotid, tonsil, pharynx, submandibular node, mycotic aneurysm of the abdominal aorta, and adrenal gland. Parotitis has been reported in children in some regions that may progress to abscess formation. Superficial organs can be best imaged with ultrasound, and MRI can be done in equivocal cases. Imaging features of these involved sites are also non-specific.

MELIOIDOSIS MIMICS

The most common mimicker of melioidosis is TB. It is difficult to differentiate between melioidosis and TB, especially in regions endemic to both diseases. Both could present similarly in many clinical conditions such as pulmonary involvement, single or multiple organ abscesses, spondylitis, and brain involvement. At times other pyogenic infections also may mimic melioidosis.

Although upper-lobe predominance is seen in both TB and melioidosis, lung apex is relatively spared in melioidosis; necrotic mediastinal lymphadenopathy is very rare in melioidosis, whereas it is commonly seen in TB. Pericarditis is rare in melioidosis. Tubercular splenic abscess is common in immunocompromised patients due to AIDS; it is rarely seen in immunocompetent patients.[15] In the brain, melioidosis abscess is typically seen as micro-abscesses. Extension along the white matter tracts and involvement of the trigeminal nerve favours a diagnosis of neuromelioidosis.

Abdominal ultrasonography is a cost-effective, non-invasive imaging modality for screening the abdomen in a suspected case of melioidosis. A CT scan has the advantage of imaging the entire abdomen and thorax simultaneously to rule out the involvement of various organs such as lungs, liver, spleen, kidney, prostate, pancreas, and peritoneal cavity. In pregnant patients and children, USG is preferred because of the risk of ionizing radiation in CT scans. In a patient with CNS involvement, MRI is preferred for diagnosis as well as follow-up. MRI is also preferred in soft-tissue infection or in the detection of early osteomyelitis. A chest X-ray is usually routinely done in these patients. An X-ray is also done if there is suspicion of osteomyelitis, septic arthritis, or spondylitis.

CONCLUSIONS

Imaging plays a critical role in evaluating multi-systemic involvement, most commonly manifested as abscesses. Despite non-specific imaging features, some of the imaging findings prompt a clinical suspicion of melioidosis in patients with high-risk factors and those living in an endemic area to initiate the appropriate antibiotic therapy. Isolated splenic or concomitant splenic and hepatic abscesses appearing as multiple small, discrete, target-like lesions or large multi-loculated lesions, particularly with honeycomb morphology in the liver and spleen, are more common in melioidosis than other infections.

REFERENCES

1. Currie BJ, et al. The Epidemiology and Clinical Spectrum of Melioidosis: 540 Cases from the 20 Year Darwin Prospective Study. PLoS Negl Trop Dis 2010; 4(11): e900.
2. Wiersinga WJ, et al. Melioidosis. N Engl J Med 2012; 367(11): 1035–44.
3. Limmathurotsakul D, et al. Predicted Global Distribution of *Burkholderia pseudomallei* and Burden of Melioidosis. Nat Microbiol 2016; 1(1): 15008.
4. Vidyalakshmi K, et al. Emerging Clinico-Epidemiological Trends in Melioidosis: Analysis of 95 Cases from Western Coastal India. Int J Infect Dis 2012; 16(7): e491–e7.
5. Lam NH, et al. Cavitary Lung Disease in Hospitalized Patients: Differences between Melioidosis and Tuberculosis. Trop Doct 2022; 52(3): 427–30. https://doi.org/10.1177/00494755221095711.
6. Lim KS, et al. Radiological Manifestations of Melioidosis. Clin Radiol 2010; 65(1): 66–72.
7. Ong SCL, et al. Honeycomb and Necklace Signs in Liver Abscesses Secondary to Melioidosis. BMJ Case Rep 2017; 2017: bcr2017222342.
8. Apisarnthanarak A, et al. Computed Tomography Characteristics of *Burkholderia pseudomallei* Liver Abscess. Clin Infect Dis 2006; 42(7): 989–93.
9. Chong VH, et al. Pancreatic Involvement in Melioidosis. Jop 2010; 11(4): 365–8.
10. Koshy M, et al. Genitourinary Melioidosis: A Descriptive Study. Trop Doct 2019; 49(2): 104–07.
11. Currie BJ, et al. Neurological Melioidosis. Acta Trop 2000; 74(2–3): 145–51.
12. Hsu CC, et al. Neuromelioidosis: Craniospinal MRI Findings in *Burkholderia pseudomallei* Infection. J Neuroimaging 2016; 26(1): 75–82.
13. Pui MH, et al. Musculoskeletal Melioidosis: Clinical and Imaging Features. Skeletal Radiol 1995; 24(7): 499–503.
14. Pattamapaspong N, et al. Musculoskeletal Melioidosis. Semin Musculoskelet Radiol 2011; 15(5): 480–8.
15. Sahoo S, et al. Tuberculous Splenic Abscess in the Immunocompetent Host: A Report and Review of Literature. Monaldi Arch Chest Dis 2020; 90(1). https://doi.org/10.4081/monaldi.2020.1167.

Diagnostic Interventional Procedures in Melioidosis

8

Sourin Bhuniya

Department of Pulmonary Medicine and Critical Care,
All India Institute of Medical Sciences, Bhubaneswar, India

Contents

INTRODUCTION

Melioidosis caused by *B. pseudomallei* in tropical countries has a mortality rate of 10–50%.[1] This high case fatality rate is mostly due to a combination of factors, including (a) lack of awareness among physicians regarding the disease, (b) resemblance to other chronic infective and non-infective conditions like tuberculosis, fungus, and malignancy, (c) difficulty and delay in diagnosis, and (d) ineffectiveness of the common antibiotics used in bacterial sepsis against the organism.[2] The diagnostic delay is primarily because of the low sensitivity of culture and difficulty in obtaining samples from sites that are often deep-seated and difficult to access. Isolation of *B. pseudomallei*

DOI: 10.1201/9781003324010-8

from blood, respiratory specimens, abscess aspirates, body fluids, or any other clinical specimen is considered the 'gold standard' for diagnosis of melioidosis.[3] Obtaining such clinical specimens frequently requires the help of minimally invasive diagnostic interventions such as flexible bronchoscopy, endobronchial ultrasound (EBUS)-guided fine-needle aspiration cytology (FNAC), and image-guided aspiration or biopsy from the difficult to reach sites.

ROLE OF FLEXIBLE BRONCHOSCOPY

Melioidosis most commonly affects the lungs, and pneumonia is the most common presentation. Other frequently reported thoracic presentations include bilateral pulmonary infiltrates, lung abscess or cavitary lesions, parapneumonic effusion, empyema, pulmonary mass, mediastinal lymphadenopathy, or mass-like lesions.[1,4] Such a spectrum of thoracic presentation is frequently misdiagnosed as tuberculosis or malignancy, especially in highly prevalent areas. Flexible bronchoscopy is a minimally invasive diagnostic tool that has often helped clinch the diagnosis of melioidosis in such scenarios. Commonly performed bronchoscopy-guided procedures such as bronchoalveolar lavage (BAL), transbronchial needle aspiration (TBNA), and transbronchial biopsy from the target sites usually help in establishing a definitive diagnosis after microbiological, cytological, and histopathological examination of the acquired specimen. Such specimens obtained by experienced bronchoscopists can provide a high yield of definitive microbiological diagnosis because the chances of such specimens becoming contaminated are minimal. Though large-scale studies on the role of bronchoscopy in the diagnosis of melioidosis are lacking, numerous reports from highly prevalent countries have shown bronchoscopy to be very useful in establishing a prompt diagnosis in cases of thoracic melioidosis with diagnostic dilemmas.[5–7]

ROLE OF EBUS-GUIDED TBNA

Timely diagnosis of melioidosis can pose a real challenge when patients present with an isolated peripheral lung nodule, mass, or mediastinal lymphadenopathy. In one of the largest prospective series from Australia, lymph node involvement was found in 2% and mediastinal mass lesion in 3% of melioidosis cases.[4] Acquiring a diagnostic sample from such a lesion would require the guidance of EBUS either with a radial or convex probe, depending upon the location of the lesion. EBUS-guided TBNA is a safe and minimally invasive procedure with very high sensitivity and specificity in evaluating mediastinal lymphadenopathy.[8,9] In patients with melioidosis presenting with mediastinal lymphadenopathy, contrast-enhanced computed tomography (CECT) of thorax and EBUS usually shows heterogeneous echo texture and areas of coagulation necrosis in the lymph nodes, which is quite similar to the features of tuberculous nodes (Figures 8.1 and 8.2).

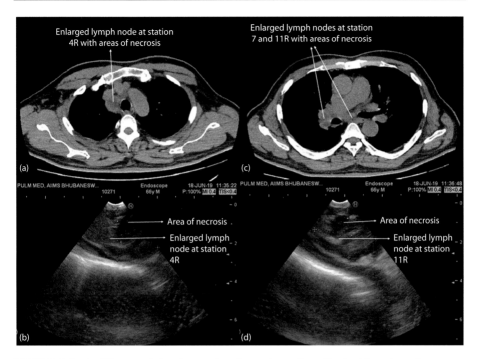

FIGURE 8.1 A CT scan of the thorax showing enlarged mediastinal lymph nodes at station 4R (A), 7 and 11R (C) with areas of necrosis as shown by arrows. EBUS images showing heterogenous echotexture and coagulation necrosis in station 4R (B) and 11R (D) nodes of the same patient.

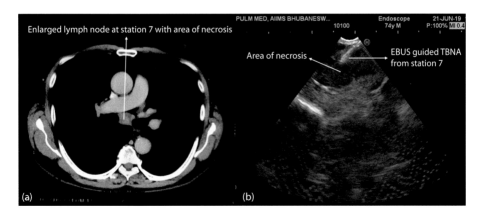

FIGURE 8.2 A CT thorax image of enlarged sub-carinal lymph node (station 7) with area of necrosis (A). The EBUS image of the same node with the TBNA needle in-situ as shown by the arrow (B).

EBUS-guided aspirate from such lesions, when subjected to cytological examination, culture, or rapid antigen test, can provide a quick diagnosis and help in the early initiation of appropriate treatment.[10] The radial probe EBUS-guided sheath technique allows very good visualization of peripheral lung lesions up to sixth or seventh order bronchus and accurate sampling from such lesions with minimal risks, as compared to conventional transbronchial biopsy under fluoroscopy guidance.[11] The diagnostic yield is usually higher than the traditional transbronchial biopsy under fluoroscopy (73% versus 14–63%, respectively).[12,13] It is worthwhile to send the EBUS-TBNA samples for bacterial cultures also, in addition to the usual histopathology and tuberculosis studies, especially from necrotic lymph nodes in diabetic patients, keeping a high index of suspicion for melioidosis. The utility of EBUS in difficult-to-diagnose cases of melioidosis has been demonstrated by various reports and case series from the high prevalent countries.[10,11,14]

ROLE OF INTERVENTIONAL RADIOLOGY AND OTHER MINIMALLY INVASIVE PROCEDURES

Melioidosis frequently presents with disseminated foci of abscesses involving different visceral organs, and microbiologically confirming *B. pseudomallei* in the clinical specimens from such extra-thoracic affected sites remains the mainstay of diagnosis.[3] Usually, this requires computed tomography (CT) or ultrasonography (USG)-guided fine-needle aspiration (FNA) of pus and tissue samples from the various body sites, such as mediastinal lymph nodes, spleen, and prostate, to establish the diagnosis.[15–17] These are minimally invasive interventions that may be particularly helpful for difficult-to-access sites or when a surgical biopsy is not possible or unavailable in resource-limited settings.[18] Among the internal organ abscesses in melioidosis, the prostate has been found to be the most commonly affected among males, especially in Australia, whereas overall, the spleen, kidney, and liver are the most commonly affected sites.[3,4] CT or USG-guided aspiration from such lesions, when coupled with rapid antigen detection tests or polymerase chain reaction (PCR)-based tests for melioidosis, can yield a quick diagnosis.[3] More specialized interventions such as trans-rectal USG-guided sextant prostate biopsy to diagnose melioidosis and drainage of melioidotic prostatic abscess by transurethral resection to eradicate persistent focus of infection have been reported.[19] In a large retrospective cohort of 153 patients over 10 years from a tertiary-level hospital in India, various interventional radiological procedures, including abscess drainage by USG-guided pig tailing and aspirations, were commonly performed (32.5%), followed by incision and drainage of peripheral soft tissue abscesses (31.2%) and orthopedic procedures such as open drainage for septic arthritis (20.8%), in the management of disseminated melioidosis infection.[20]

Unlike in adults, involvement of cervical lymph nodes and salivary glands by *B. pseudomallei* is quite common in children, especially in Southeast Asian countries. Melioidosis may also present with suppurative parotitis in about 40% of children in this region, but it is extremely rare in Australia.[21,22] A high index of suspicion of melioidosis is warranted in children presenting with cervical lymphadenopathy and an occult splenic abscess or associated with pneumonia or septic arthritis in high prevalent regions. Consideration of FNA from cervical lymph nodes followed by microbiological confirmation in such cases has been found to clinch the diagnosis in around 75% of children.[21]

SURGERY IN MELIOIDOSIS

Rarely has surgery been shown to establish the diagnosis of melioidosis or manage its unwanted complications. Video-assisted thoracoscopy and mini-thoracotomy have been shown to help diagnose a patient presenting with right superior mediastinal mass lesion, where even bronchoscopy or endoscopy-guided FNA biopsy could not yield a definitive diagnosis.[23] Splenectomy has also been performed as an uncommon procedure for the management of melioidotic abscesses.[20] Melioidosis is known to cause mycotic aneurysm, a rare but dreaded complication in about 1% of affected patients, requiring prompt consideration of surgical intervention and prolonged appropriate antibiotic therapy.[24] Early consideration of surgical interventions, wherever indicated, improves the clinical outcome and reduces mortality.[20]

Diagnosis of *B. pseudomallei* with its protean manifestations has been a big challenge in the resource-limited settings of Southeast Asian countries. Awareness about the disease among primary care physicians, a high index of suspicion, and prompt referral of suspected cases to higher centres, with all the appropriate diagnostic facilities, are the keys to early diagnosis and preventing mortality from this tropical infection.

REFERENCES

1. Cheng AC, et al. Melioidosis: Epidemiology, Pathophysiology, and Management. Clin Microbiol Rev 2005; 18(2): 383–416.
2. Wiersinga WJ, et al. Melioidosis. Nat Rev Dis Primers 2018; 4: 17107.
3. Kingsley PV, et al. Pitfalls and Optimal Approaches to Diagnose Melioidosis. Asian Pac J Trop Med 2016; 9(6): 515–24.
4. Currie BJ, et al. The Epidemiology and Clinical Spectrum of Melioidosis: 540 Cases from the 20 Year Darwin Prospective Study. PLoS Negl Trop Dis 2010; 4(11): e900.
5. Gulati U, et al. Case Report: A Fatal Case of Latent Melioidosis Activated by COVID-19. Am J Trop Med Hyg 2022;106(4): 1170–72.
6. Lee SW, et al. A Case of Melioidosis Presenting as Migrating Pulmonary Infiltration: The First Case in Korea. J Korean Med Sci 2005; 20(1): 139–42.
7. Kho SS, et al. Mediastinal Melioidosis Masquerading as Malignancy of the Lung. Lancet 2021; 397(10278): e8.
8. Gu P, et al. Endobronchial Ultrasound-Guided Transbronchial Needle Aspiration for Staging of Lung Cancer: A Systematic Review and Meta-Analysis. Eur J Cancer 2009; 45(8): 1389–96.
9. Casadio C, et al. Molecular Testing for Targeted Therapy in Advanced Non-Small Cell Lung Cancer: Suitability of Endobronchial Ultrasound Transbronchial Needle Aspiration. Am J Clin Pathol 2015; 144(4): 629–34.

10. Rahman KKM, et al. Utility of Endobronchial Ultrasound Guided Trans-Bronchial Needle Aspiration in Diagnosis of Melioidosis - Case Series and Review of Literature. Monaldi Arch Chest Dis 2020; 90(3): 420–24.
11. Zaw KK, et al. Chronic Pulmonary Melioidosis Masquerading as Lung Malignancy Diagnosed by EBUS Guided Sheath Technique. Respir Med Case Rep 2019; 28: 100894.
12. Baaklini WA, et al. Diagnostic Yield of Fiberoptic Bronchoscopy in Evaluating Solitary Pulmonary Nodules. Chest 2000; 117(4): 1049–54.
13. Wang Memoli JS, et al. Meta-Analysis of Guided Bronchoscopy for the Evaluation of the Pulmonary Nodule. Chest 2012; 142(2): 385–93.
14. Chan HP, et al. Mediastinal Lymphadenopathy: Melioidosis Mimicking Tuberculosis. Trop Med Health 2015; 43(2): 93–4.
15. Arzola JM, et al. A Case of Prostatitis Due to *Burkholderia pseudomallei*. Nat Clin Pract Urol 2007; 4(2): 111–4.
16. Lin CY, et al. Melioidosis Presenting with Isolated Splenic Abscesses: A Case Report. Kaohsiung J Med Sci 2007; 23(8): 417–21.
17. Truong KK, et al. Case of a Lung Mass Due to Melioidosis in Mexico. Am J Case Rep 2015; 16: 272–5.
18. Sher-Locketz C, et al. Successful Introduction of Fine Needle Aspiration Biopsy for Diagnosis of Pediatric Lymphadenopathy. Pediatr Infect Dis J 2017; 36(8): 811–14.
19. Yip SK, et al. Clinics in Diagnostic Imaging (57). Melioidotic Prostatic Abscess. Singapore Med J 2001; 42(1): 41–3.
20. George AJ, et al. Surgical Management of Melioidosis: 10-Year Retrospective Data from a Tertiary Hospital in India. Int J Med Rev Case Rep 2020; 4(6): 34–37.
21. Mohan A, et al. Fine-Needle Aspiration to Improve Diagnosis of Melioidosis of the Head and Neck in Children: A Study from Sarawak, Malaysia. BMC Infect Dis 2021; 21(1): 1069.
22. Wiersinga WJ, et al. Melioidosis. N Engl J Med 2012; 367(11): 1035–44.
23. Ashraf O, et al. Thoracic Melioidosis: A Diagnostic Dilemma. Asian Cardiovasc Thorac Ann 2015; 23(2): 219–20.
24. Li PH, et al. Melioidosis Mycotic Aneurysm: An Uncommon Complication of an Uncommon Disease. Respir Med Case Rep 2015; 14: 43–6.

Drug Management of Melioidosis

9

Prasanta R Mohapatra

Department of Pulmonary Medicine and Critical Care,
All India Institute of Medical Sciences, Bhubaneswar, India

Contents

INTRODUCTION

Melioidosis is caused by the Gram-negative bacterium *Burkholderia pseudomallei*, manifested as pneumonia, bacteremia, multiple organ abscesses, localized skin lesion, septic arthritis, osteomyelitis, and severe sepsis. The treatment is prolonged with initial intensive phases of antibiotics in acute melioidosis, followed by eradication of dormant bacilli. The Darwin melioidosis guideline, described as a new treatment paradigm, has been associated with relatively low rates of recrudescence and relapse.

The earlier treatment for managing melioidosis was a combination of three drugs, cotrimoxazole, chloramphenicol, and doxycycline, with a lower success rate. In some places, the injection of kanamycin was used as the fourth drug in combination.[1] The overall mortality rate until that time for bacteremic patients was as high as 87%.[2] 1989 was an important year for the introduction of ceftazidime, which dramatically improved disease and halved the risk of melioidosis death from 74% to 37%.[3,4] The dose used for ceftazidime (120 mg/kg of body weight/day). Carbapenems, like meropenem and imipenem, have the greatest *in vitro* activity against *B. pseudomallei*.[5]

Burkholderia pseudomallei has broad intrinsic antimicrobial resistance to some antibiotics, and long-term treatment consists of an intensive intravenous phase of a minimum

DOI: 10.1201/9781003324010-9

81

of 2 weeks with ceftazidime, meropenem, or imipenem, which is to be followed by an oral eradication phase of at least 12 weeks, usually with trimethoprim-sulfamethoxazole is essential for cure.[6] The recommended duration of intravenous therapy is determined by the disease site and severity of melioidosis.[7] Ceftazidime is commonly used for most cases, with meropenem usually kept for the severe disease requiring ICU admission. Oral trimethoprim-sulfamethoxazole is added during intensive phase therapy in cutaneous melioidosis, osteomyelitis or septic arthritis, central nervous system (CNS) infection, and deep-seated collections.[7] The rationale for double oral and intravenous treatment is to increase tissue penetration and to limit the emergence of resistance. Current therapy guidelines of the Royal Darwin Hospital recommend an initial intensive phase followed by an eradication phase (Table 9.1).[6] This treatment guideline has evolved over two decades, with more than 1150 successive subjects of culture-proven melioidosis.

In the resource constraint areas where prolonged intravenous therapy may not be affordable, at least 10 days of intravenous therapy is recommended.[8] The duration of oral eradication therapy is the key determinant of relapse.[6]

Recrudescence is defined as 'the development of clinical illness during the oral eradication phase with a concurrent new culture of *B. pseudomallei* in a clinical specimen'.[6]

Recurrence is defined as 'the development of clinical illness **after** the oral eradication phase, with a new culture of *B. pseudomallei* in a clinical specimen'. Recurrence can be either relapse with a previous genotype or a new *B. pseudomallei* with a different genotype.[6]

CLINICIANS' CONCERNS

The optimal duration of intravenous therapy has been a matter of concern. The latest 2020 Royal Darwin Hospital guideline has contributed to reducing rates of recrudescence and relapse in their region and a clear decline in mortality.

The revised Royal Darwin Hospital guideline recommends an intravenous dose of ceftazidime at 50 mg/kg of body weight (up to 2 g) every 6 to 8 hours if the patient is on the ward or meropenem at 25 mg/kg (up to 1 g) every 8 hours if in the ICU during the intensive phase.[6]

The duration of 2 weeks is for an uncomplicated infection. A minimum of 4 weeks of intravenous antibiotics should be given with positive blood cultures suffering from pneumonia with ICU admission, lymphadenopathy, or multi-lobar unilateral or bilateral pneumonia.[6] A minimum of 6 weeks should be given in deep-seated abscess collection, which is defined as 'abscess anywhere other than skin, lungs, bone, CNS, or vasculature'.[6] A minimum of 4 weeks of intravenous antibiotics should be given with positive blood cultures suffering from pneumonia with ICU admission, or with lymphadenopathy or multi-lobar unilateral or bilateral pneumonia.[6] A minimum duration of 8 weeks is necessary for arterial infection or neurological melioidosis.[6]

The oral eradication phase is an integral part of therapy with cotrimoxazole dose, depending on weight and age, ranging from 36 months. Dosage recommendations for adults include the following: for the weight of 40 kg, 160/800 mg every 12 hours;

TABLE 9.1   2020 Revised Darwin melioidosis guideline[6]

ANTIBIOTIC DURATION DETERMINING FOCUS	MINIMUM INTENSIVE PHASE DURATION (WEEKS)[a]	ERADICATION PHASE DURATION (MONTHS)[f]
Skin abscess	2	3
Bacteraemia with no focus	2	3
Unilateral unilobar pneumonia without lymphadenopathy[b], ICU admission, and with negative blood cultures	2	3
Multi-lobar unilateral or bilateral pneumonia without lymphadenopathy[b], ICU admission, and with negative blood cultures OR Unilateral unilobar pneumonia without lymphadenopathy[b], ICU admission, but with positive blood cultures	3	3
Pneumonia with either lymphadenopathy[b] or ICU admission OR Multi-lobar unilateral or bilateral pneumonia with positive blood cultures	4	3
Deep-seated collection[c]	4[d]	3
Osteomyelites	6	6
Central nervous system infection	8	6
Arterial infection[e]	8[d]	6[g]

[a] Clinical judgment to guide prolongation of intensive phase if the improvement is slow or if blood cultures remain positive at 7 days.
[b] Defined as enlargement of any hilar or mediastinal lymph node to greater than 10 mm in diameter.
[c] Defined as an abscess anywhere other than skin, lungs, bone, CNS, or vasculature. Septic arthritis is considered a deep-seated collection.
[d] Intensive phase duration is timed from the date of the most recent drainage or resection where culture of the drainage specimen or resected material grew *B. pseudomallei* or where no specimen was sent for culture; the clock is not reset if the specimen is culture-negative.
[e] Most commonly presenting as mycotic aneurysm.
[f] If concurrent oral therapy is not indicated in the intensive phase, oral eradication therapy is to commence at the start of the final week of planned intensive intravenous therapy, with the timing of eradication duration commencing from the day after the last intravenous therapy.
[g] Life-long suppressive antibiotic therapy may be required following vascular prosthetic surgery.
Source: Reproduced with permission under Creative Commons Attribution license (CC BY), from PLOS Neglected Tropical Diseases, https://doi.org/10.1371/journal.pntd.0008659.[6]

40–60 kg, 240/1200 mg every 12 hours; and for above 60 kg weight, 320/1600 mg every 12 hours.[6]

Although TMP-SMX is thought to be a bacteriostatic antimicrobial with time-dependent action, a time-kill study has shown the target *in vivo* drug concentrations with the bactericidal effect, which is concentration-dependent.[9] Oral doxycycline and amoxicillin-clavulanic acid are used as second-line drugs. The recommended amoxicillin-clavulanic acid dosage is 20/5 mg per kilogram of body weight three times daily.[10] The relapses were more common in patients with severe disease than those with localized melioidosis in a large study in Thailand.[11] Clinicians may prolong the duration of intravenous therapy when there is an apprehension of intolerance to cotrimoxazole eradication therapy[12] and the use of doxycycline as second-line oral eradication therapy.[6]

The clinical trial also showed that maintenance therapy duration is critical, particularly with patients receiving less than 12 weeks of treatment having a 5.7-fold-increased risk of relapse or death.[13] Some evidence has shown the non-inferiority and improved tolerability when comparing cotrimoxazole (TMP-SMX) alone and cotrimoxazole with doxycycline.[14] Other research in Australia has revealed decreased rates of relapse or recrudescence depending on the duration of intensive-phase therapy.[7] With a median intensive phase of 26 days, the relapse or recrudescence rate decreased from 5.2% to 0.5%, irrespective of compliance to the eradication/oral phase.[7] Therefore, the optimal dose and duration are critical for the relapse or recrudescence of melioidosis.

Current Darwin guidelines recommend a minimum intensive phase of 2 weeks for skin abscess bacteremia with no focus, unilateral unilobar pneumonia without lymphadenopathy, even with admission to intensive care unit but with negative blood cultures skin abscess, bacteremia without focus, and pneumonia without lymphadenopathy or ICU admission. Four weeks is required for pneumonia with lymphadenopathy or ICU admission or deep-seated collection (abscess anywhere other than skin), 6 weeks for osteomyelitis, and 8 weeks for CNS or arterial infection.[7] The study alters traditional thinking that choice and duration of eradication therapy are the most important predictors of relapse.[7] Further analysis of septic arthritis and osteomyelitis management suggests that 5 weeks of intravenous therapy or 4 weeks for an isolated single joint without osteomyelitis will suffice. Source control is an important feature in overall management.[2]

The majority of visceral abscesses, other than prostatic, responded to antimicrobial therapy alone in one study; prostatic abscesses greater than 1 cm should be considered for drainage.[15,16] Fever clearance may be slow, with a median of 9 days in one study, and therefore, this may not necessarily stand as an indication for surgical intervention.[15]

While ideal, source control may not be achieved in every circumstance, particularly in resource-limited settings. It is important to note that treatment success has been achieved with prolonged therapy in the setting of difficult to drain abscesses.[16,17]

B. pseudomallei strains also shown to be having multi-drug resistant against meropenem, imipenem, and ceftazidime.[18] *B. pseudomallei* is also susceptible to amoxicillin-clavulanic acid, and intravenous and oral preparations may be used as a second-line agent in patients intolerant to TMP-SMX or with sulfonamide allergy, or where other agents may be contraindicated due to pregnancy or young age.[10]

CONCLUSION

The management of septicaemic melioidosis has been mentioned in Chapter 13 of this book. New siderophore cephalosporin **cefiderocol** is highly active *in vitro* against *B. pseudomallei* primary clinical isolates. However, resistance has been detected in a smaller number of isolates.[19] **Finafloxacin**, a fifth-generation fluoroquinolone, may be useful in the coming days as a part of combination treatment for melioidosis.[20]

Still, in patients on treatment, variant selection and acquired resistance driven by mutations in *B. pseudomallei* can develop through various mechanisms that need to be elucidated continuously.

REFERENCES

1. Leelarasamee A, et al. Melioidosis: Review and Update. Rev Infect Dis 1989; 11(3): 413–25.
2. Dance D. Treatment and Prophylaxis of Melioidosis. Int J Antimicrob Agents 2014; 43(4): 310–8.
3. White NJ, et al. Halving of Mortality of Severe Melioidosis by Ceftazidime. Lancet 1989; 2(8665): 697–701.
4. Jayanetra P, et al. *Pseudomonas pseudomallei*: 1. Infection in Thailand. Southeast Asian J Trop Med Public Health 1974; 5(4): 487–91.
5. Smith MD, et al. In-Vitro Activity of Carbapenem Antibiotics Against Beta-Lactam Susceptible and Resistant Strains of *Burkholderia pseudomallei*. J Antimicrob Chemother 1996; 37(3): 611–5.
6. Sullivan RP, et al. 2020 Review and Revision of the 2015 Darwin Melioidosis Treatment Guideline; Paradigm Drift Not Shift. PLoS Negl Trop Dis 2020; 14(9): e0008659.
7. Pitman MC, et al. Intravenous Therapy Duration and Outcomes in Melioidosis: A New Treatment Paradigm. PLoS Negl Trop Dis 2015; 9(3): e0003586.
8. Wiersinga WJ, et al. Melioidosis. Nat Rev Dis Primers 2018; 4: 17107.
9. Cheng AC, et al. Dosing Regimens of Cotrimoxazole (Trimethoprim-Sulfamethoxazole) for Melioidosis. Antimicrob Agents Chemother 2009; 53(10): 4193–9.
10. Cheng AC, et al. Consensus Guidelines for Dosing of Amoxicillin-Clavulanate in Melioidosis. Am J Trop Med Hyg 2008; 78(2): 208–9.
11. Chaowagul W, et al. Relapse in Melioidosis: Incidence and Risk Factors. J Infect Dis 1993; 168(5): 1181–5.
12. Sullivan RP, et al. Oral Eradication Therapy for Melioidosis: Important but Not Without Risks. Int J Infect Dis 2019; 80: 111–14.
13. Chaowagul W, et al. Open-Label Randomized Trial of Oral Trimethoprim-Sulfamethoxazole, Doxycycline, and Chloramphenicol Compared with Trimethoprim-Sulfamethoxazole and Doxycycline for Maintenance Therapy of Melioidosis. Antimicrob Agents Chemother 2005; 49(10): 4020–5.
14. Chetchotisakd P, et al. Trimethoprim-Sulfamethoxazole Versus Trimethoprim-Sulfamethoxazole Plus Doxycycline as Oral Eradicative Treatment for Melioidosis (MERTH): A Multicentre, Double-Blind, Non-Inferiority, Randomised Controlled Trial. Lancet 2014; 383(9919): 807–14.
15. Currie BJ, et al. Endemic Melioidosis in Tropical Northern Australia: A 10-Year Prospective Study and Review of the Literature. Clin Infect Dis 2000; 31(4): 981–6.
16. Morse LP, et al. Prostatic Abscess Due to *Burkholderia pseudomallei*: 81 Cases from a 19-Year Prospective Melioidosis Study. J Urol 2009; 182(2): 542–7; discussion 47.
17. Currie BJ, et al. The Epidemiology and Clinical Spectrum of Melioidosis: 540 Cases from the 20 Year Darwin Prospective Study. PLoS Negl Trop Dis 2010; 4(11): e900.
18. Schnetterle M, et al. Genomic and RT-qPCR Analysis of Trimethoprim-Sulfamethoxazole and Meropenem Resistance in *Burkholderia pseudomallei* Clinical Isolates. PLoS Negl Trop Dis 2021; 15(2): e0008913.

19. Burnard D, et al. *Burkholderia pseudomallei* Clinical Isolates Are Highly Susceptible *In Vitro* to Cefiderocol, a Siderophore Cephalosporin. Antimicrob Agents Chemother 2021; 65(2): e00685–e20.
20. Barnes KB, et al. Investigation of a Combination Therapy Approach for the Treatment of Melioidosis. Front Microbiol 2022; 13: 934312.

Management of Melioidosis

A Surgeon's Perspective

10

Prakash K Sasmal

Department of Surgery, All India Institute of Medical Sciences, Bhubaneswar, India

Pankaj Kumar

Department of Surgery, All India Institute of Medical Sciences, Bhubaneswar, India

Contents

INTRODUCTION

Melioidosis, also known as Whitmore's disease, an infectious disease caused by the Gram-negative bacillus *Burkholderia pseudomallei*, is increasingly being reported

DOI: 10.1201/9781003324010-10

in India, causing a broad spectrum of clinical presentations, including pneumonia, cutaneous/parietal abscesses, genitourinary tract infections, parotid gland, lymph nodes, septic arthritis, osteomyelitis, and various intra-abdominal organ abscesses including liver, spleen, pancreas, etc.[1] There are few reports from India regarding the isolates of the bacillus in the soil of the eastern and western coastal belts including few southern states, thus, stressing the fact that they are related to the local environment.[2] The portal of entry of the bacillus is through the airway, broken skin, and possible ingestion.[3]

The risk factors identified are diabetes mellitus, renal disease, haematological diseases, chronic lung disease, frequent alcohol intake, occupational exposure to soil and surface water, elderly, and immunosuppression.[2] In a retrospective study of 153 patients from India diagnosed with melioidosis, the most common risk factor was type 2 diabetes mellitus found in 107 patients (68.6%). Chronic lung diseases and alcohol abuse were other relative risk factors.[3]

A wide array of clinical presentations is reported in melioidosis, ranging from asymptomatic infection, acute fulminant sepsis, and subacute multi-focal abscesses to mild chronic disease.[4] An asymptomatic infection, also termed latent melioidosis, can later develop into active disease intermittently after the initial infection.[5] A surgeon often encounters patients with cutaneous abscesses, abscesses of the parotid gland, lung, liver, spleen, prostate, etc., as routine surgical cases. It is only with a high index of suspicion and on the microbiological assay that melioidosis is confirmed. The typical presentation of melioidosis to a surgeon is with an abscess and often with sepsis. Hence, prompt diagnosis and initiation of treatment, both medical and surgical, can reduce mortality.[6] Our first experience of melioidosis was with a middle-aged male with a ruptured splenic abscess with sepsis. The retrospective study by George et al. from India found septic arthritis/bone involvement to be the most common presentation, followed by intra-abdominal abscesses.[3]

Once confirmed through culture, the surgical management of melioidosis at different sites is based on the risk factors present in the patient along with the general condition. The mortality from melioidosis is very high, ranging from 15% to 25%.[7] Surgical intervention is required in many patients, depending on the site of involvement. In the retrospective study by George et al., they reported surgical intervention in 50% of the patients with melioidosis.[3] They have also highlighted the increased mortality rates when surgical intervention is performed in patients suffering from melioidosis with bacteraemia and sepsis. The possible reasons could be delayed diagnosis, poor general condition of the patient, usually with severe sepsis, and in ICU on a ventilator, often with ionotropic supports.[3]

The main line of treatment for melioidosis is specific antimicrobials guided by the Darwin melioidosis treatment guideline comprising intravenous ceftazidime, meropenem, or imipenem in the intensive phase for 2 weeks followed by an oral eradication phase of at least 12 weeks, usually with trimethoprim-sulfamethoxazole.[8,9] However, the surgeon often encounters patients with ruptured abscesses in various solid organs. Surgical drainage of the pus, suspected due to melioidosis, is required and feasible in large, single, and localized abscesses.[10] The various intervention options reported for different organ systems found in the existing literature will be discussed.

GASTROINTESTINAL MELIOIDOSIS

The common intra-abdominal organs involved in melioidosis are the spleen, liver, and pancreas, manifesting as abscesses or infected pancreatic collections.[11] The most common abdominal organ affected is the spleen, followed by the liver causing hepato-splenic abscesses.[12] Most cases can be managed by ultrasound-guided percutaneous catheter drainage (PCD) of the abscess and antibiotics (ceftazidime and cotrimoxa-zole).[11] Pancreatic involvement in melioidosis presents either with multi-focal micro-abscesses or focal collection.[9] Most cases of pancreatic abscesses are part of the multiple organ involvement with multi-focal micro-abscesses managed by antibiotics.[10] However, in post-pancreatitis secondary abscess with melioidosis, surgical interventions like debridement[13] or radio-guided percutaneous drainage may be required.

Our first experience with melioidosis started with a middle-aged male farmer, a chronic alcoholic with a ruptured splenic abscess presenting with fever for a month and systemic signs of sepsis (Figure 10.1). One of the abscesses ruptured but was well contained and did not directly communicate with the peritoneal cavity. The operative procedure was complicated because of dense peri-splenic adhesions from peri-splenitis as sequelae of ruptured splenic abscess (Figure 10.2). The patient succumbed in the postoperative period due to acute fulminant septicaemia with multi-organ failure following melioidosis.[14] In the literature review, the mortality rates from melioidosis worldwide are very high, from 15% to 25%.[7] Hence, it is prudent to stress early diagnosis and treatment to reduce the morbidity and mortality rate. The outcomes of patients with gastro-intestinal melioidosis are good following surgical interventions. However, the mortality rate is significant in those patients with bacteraemia and sepsis, where surgical interventions are less likely to be performed.[7] There are few reports on the surgical excision of the spleen followed by anti-infection therapy for melioidosis with a good outcome.[6,7] Pancreatic melioidosis can mimic a localized or diffuse malignancy on computerized tomography (CT) imaging, which can be ascertained by tissue sampling.[10] A few cases

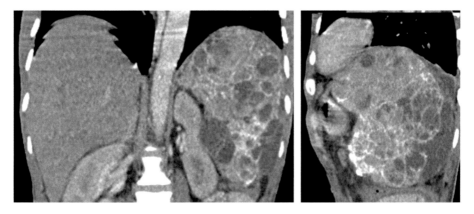

FIGURE 10.1   The CT scan of the abdomen shows a splenic abscess.

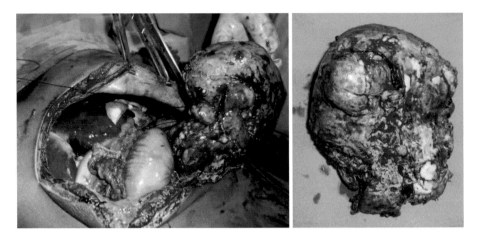

FIGURE 10.2   An operative specimen of a spleen showing multiple abscesses.

of splenic abscesses with splenic vein thrombosis are reported, which are rare and managed by antibiotics alone.[15]

A report from India highlighted melioidosis affecting the small intestine, manifesting as perforation and acute abdomen.[16] The patient was managed by omental patch closure of the perforations and a thorough lavage of the abdomen along with imipenem and doxycycline for 14 days, followed by cotrimoxazole (160 +800 mg) for 4 months.[16]

A case report by Sugi Subramaniam et al. from India reported intra-abdominal melioidosis affecting the omentum and manifesting as an intra-abdominal abscess sensitive to ceftazidime and ciprofloxacin.[17] The disease masqueraded as peritoneal tuberculosis. The patient, however, succumbed on post-operative day 5 due to septic shock.[17]

In a retrospective study from Singapore, patients who underwent surgery (both open or laparoscopic) for pancreato-splenic abscess benefited from a shorter duration of antibiotics (6 weeks instead of 3 months) except in cases with synchronous infection.[18] The MEDLINE database review from 1980 to 2021 of 10 reported articles on pancreatic/splenic abscesses caused by melioidosis showed conservative management failed in all the cases and required surgical interventions in the form of splenectomy.[18] A unique case from India reported a lesser sac hematoma after rupture of the mycotic aneurysm from the splenic artery involving the gastric wall and multiple splenic abscesses. CT-guided aspiration of the abscess and culture revealed *Burkholderia pseudomallei*. Even after medical management with intravenous ceftazidime 1 gm intravenous (IV) and tablet sulphamethoxazole+ trimethoprim twice daily for 2 weeks, the patient had to undergo surgical evacuation of the large lesser sac haematoma, suture repair of the posterior gastric wall erosion and splenectomy with ligation of the splenic artery proximal to aneurysm.[19]

Incidence of isolated liver abscess due to melioidosis is not very common. The liver is involved in disseminated cases and is clinically indistinguishable from other causes of liver abscesses.[20] The treatment of liver abscess due to melioidosis is mostly imaging-guided percutaneous drainage with concomitant recommended antibiotics. The authors managed a large liver abscess at segment eight, confirmed later in culture studies as melioidosis by laparoscopic guided pigtail insertion.[20]

PAROTID MELIOIDOSIS

Involvement of the parotid land commonly manifests as suppurative parotitis or abscesses. Most of the case reports on parotid abscess due to *B. pseudomallei* are from India, highlighting the importance of chlorinated drinking water.[21,22] This hypothesis may be the fact behind the rarity of parotid abscesses in Australia, where there are high rates of chlorination of water supplies.[22]

We had the experience of two consecutive young patients with parotid abscesses from the same village who presented with acute suppurative parotitis. As in a routine case, incision and drainage of the parotid abscess were done, and the diagnosis of melioidosis was confirmed only in the culture study. They responded very well to antibiotics after that. An epidemiological survey revealed their use of underground unchlorinated water for drinking purposes. It is unclear from the existing literature whether only appropriate antibiotics are sufficient for the abscess resolution or surgical drainage of the abscess to be routinely carried out.

SOFT-TISSUE ABSCESS

Melioidosis manifests as a cutaneous abscess in various sites of the body. We found cutaneous abscesses in three patients' abdominal wall, back, and scalp (Figure 10.3). Two of the patients were known diabetic on irregular treatment. It is only after incision and drainage of the abscess, as done routinely, and culture of the pus that *B. pseudomallei was* isolated. All the patients received cotrimoxazole as the eradication phase of antibiotics for the appropriate duration. It is not clear from the existing literature whether this cutaneous abscess will resolve only with antibiotics. In the review article

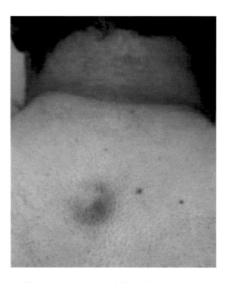

FIGURE 10.3 Soft tissue abscess on the back in a diabetic patient.

reporting cases from India, out of 85 reported cases, 84% presented as acute infections, amongst which the most common clinical presentation was soft tissue abscess (36%).[23] A case report from Malaysia presented an unusual site of melioidosis as pyomyositis with abscesses in the obturator externus and adductor muscles. The pus was surgically drained, and *B. pseudomallei* was cultured from the pus.[24]

GENITOURINARY MELIOIDOSIS

Prior reports of melioidosis have mentioned genitourinary involvement. Even though it is not widely known, genitourinary involvement considerably increases the burden of melioidosis. The organ most frequently involved is the prostate, followed by the kidney, bladder, and seminal vesicles. According to current studies, *E. coli* is the most frequent bacterium associated with chronic bacterial prostatitis; however, melioidosis should also be considered when appropriate. In northern Australia, and Southeast Asia, including India, prostatic abscesses are a common complication of *B. pseudomallei* infection (Table 10.1). Mycobacterium tuberculosis is the most frequent infectious agent causing chronic genitourinary illness in developing tropical countries. The pathogenetic mechanisms and risk factors of the two diseases share many similarities. Establishing a correct diagnosis is hampered by a lack of knowledge and limited laboratory resources. Diabetes, alcohol use, and chronic renal disease are frequently mentioned risk factors. Poor glycaemic control increases the risk significantly.

Most patients have disseminated disease (>80%). Patients are usually symptomatic for a long duration, with fever as the most common presenting symptom. The most frequently involved organ is the prostate. The kidney, bladder, and seminal vesicles are some additional organs that may be affected. The obstruction and retention symptoms should alert the clinician to this diagnosis in addition to the typical urinary system symptoms. Most patients have urinary symptoms, an abnormal prostate on examination, abnormal

TABLE 10.1   Review of literature on genitourinary melioidosis

AUTHOR	NUMBER OF CASES	YEAR OF PUBLICATION	GEOGRAPHICAL LOCATION
Morse, L.[25]	81	2009	Australia
Currie, BJ.[26]	76	2000	Australia
Chien, JM.[27]	52	2018	Singapore
Kozlowska, J.[28]	22	2018	Australia
Koshy, M.[29]	20	2019	India
Puthucheary, SD.[30]	10	1992	Malaysia
Dhiensiri, T.[31]	10	1995	Thailand
Chaowagul, W.[32]	8	1989	Thailand
Punyagupta, S.[33]	7	1989	Thailand

urinalysis results, or a positive urine culture for *B. pseudomallei*. The most frequent symptom is a positive urine culture, followed by dysuria. The most frequent findings on genitourinary tract examination are discomfort and enlargement of the prostatic gland. Less than 50% of men with melioidosis have a prostatic abscess. With minor prostatic tenderness present in fewer than 50% of patients, urinary retention is seen in almost half of the patients. Among the urinary symptoms are dysuria, urinary retention, frequency, suprapubic pain, hesitancy, nocturia, incontinence, perineal pain, urgency, rectal pain, urinary discharge, and dribbling. Other symptoms include scrotal, renal, and epididymitis abscesses. Pyelonephritis and renal abscesses are other signs of renal involvement. Some patients may display symptoms of cystitis, but because some symptoms could go unnoticed, it is advised that all male patients with melioidosis have a high level of suspicion and undergo aggressive radiological screening.

Urine and pus cultures and the necessary clinical imaging are crucial for diagnosis. Urinary leukocytes $>50 \times 106$/L have 100% sensitivity, but lack specificity (60%). Urinary erythrocytes level of $>50 \times 106$/L has sensitivity and specificity of 50% and 70%, respectively. Bacteriuria can be observed in about 75% of patients and has a specificity of more than 90%. The slight increase in prostate-specific antigen (PSA) may be explained by preferential involvement of the peripheral zone of the prostate. So, the PSA level is typically just slightly elevated. Although ultrasound (USG) is more commonly available, the false-negative rate is as high as 80%. Positron emission tomography (PET) may detect small abscesses that are invisible on CT or US. However, the clinical value of this is still debatable because such tiny abscesses might respond to antibiotic therapy without drainage. A possible advantage of PET is that, theoretically, it may be more beneficial than CT in demonstrating the clearance of an active infection.

MANAGEMENT OF GENITOURINARY MELIOIDOSIS

Patients with prostatic abscesses are treated with intravenous ceftazidime or meropenem for 2–4 weeks in the intensive intravenous phase. For those patients in whom *B. pseudomallei* could be determined, trimethoprim-sulfamethoxazole was added during the first 2 weeks of their hospitalization. The patients who completed the intensive phase are advised an oral eradication therapy with trimethoprim-sulfamethoxazole for 12 weeks.[28]

Most authors suggest drainage of prostatic abscess >10–15 mm in diameter.[25] Drainage of the abscess is necessary for patients who do not improve with conservative therapy. When drainage is recommended, transrectal ultrasound (TRUS)-guided needle aspiration or transurethral drainage is the method of choice.[25,34] The transurethral, transperineal, or transrectal routes can be used to drain persistent or sizable recurring abscesses successfully. The likelihood of needing drainage surgery increases noticeably if the patient has urinary retention. If minimally invasive treatment is unsuccessful, open surgical intervention may be required.

While larger melioidosis abscesses require drainage, smaller abscesses (less than 1 cm) can resolve with antibiotic therapy alone.[25] A systemic and localized recurrence of infection is more likely in this situation, and persistent abscesses can still harbour viable bacteria months after receiving proper and standardized antibiotic therapy. Therefore, drainage is a crucial addition to antibiotic treatment in cases of large or persistent abscesses.

CONCLUSION

Melioidosis, although it responds very well to appropriate antibiotics, still may require early surgical intervention when indicated in specific sites, which would be ideal and life-saving. As the disease is mainly confined to some regions of the world, further prospective studies on a large group of patients are essential for exploring the benefits of various treatment modalities.

REFERENCES

1. Wiersinga WJ, et al. Melioidosis. Nat Rev Dis Primers 2018; 4: 17107.
2. Princess I, et al. Melioidosis: An Emerging Infection with Fatal Outcomes. Indian J Crit Care Med 2017; 21(6): 397–400.
3. George AJ, et al. Surgical Management of Melioidosis: 10-Year Retrospective Data from a Tertiary Hospital in India. Int J Med Rev Case Rep 2020; 4(6): 34–7.
4. Chang CY. Periorbital Cellulitis and Eyelid Abscess as Ocular Manifestations of Melioidosis: A Report of Three Cases in Sarawak, Malaysian Borneo. IDCases 2020; 19: e00683.
5. Shaaban H, et al. Reactivation of Latent Melioidosis Presenting with Acute Pyelonephritis and Bacteremia. Avicenna J Med 2014; 4(1): 20–1.
6. Chen H, et al. A Case Report: Splenic Abscess Caused by *Burkholderia pseudomallei*. Med (Baltimore) 2018; 97(26): e11208.
7. Currie BJ, et al. The Epidemiology and Clinical Spectrum of Melioidosis: 540 Cases from the 20 Year Darwin Prospective Study. PLoS Negl Trop Dis 2010; 4(11): e900.
8. Saravu K, et al. Melioidosis in Southern India: Epidemiological and Clinical Profile. Southeast Asian J Trop Med Public Health 2010; 41(2): 401–9.
9. Sullivan RP, et al. 2020 Review and Revision of the 2015 Darwin Melioidosis Treatment Guideline; Paradigm Drift Not Shift. PLoS Negl Trop Dis 2020; 14(9): e0008659.
10. Chong VH, et al. Pancreatic Involvement in Melioidosis. Jop 2010; 11(4): 365–8.
11. Jagtap N, et al. Gastrointestinal Manifestations of Melioidosis: A Single Center Experience. Indian J Gastroenterol 2017; 36(2): 141–4.
12. Lim KS, et al. Radiological Manifestations of Melioidosis. Clin Radiol 2010; 65(1): 66–72.
13. Srikanth G, et al. Pancreatic Abscess: 10 Years Experience. ANZ J Surg 2002; 72(12): 881–6.
14. Behera B, et al. A Case of Fatal Septicaemic Melioidosis from Odisha. Tropical Gastroenterol Emerg Infect Dis 2017; 38: 134–7.
15. Chang CY. Ruptured Splenic Abscess and Splenic Vein Thrombosis Secondary to Melioidosis: A Case Report. J Acute Dis 2020; 9: 89–92.
16. Karuna T, et al. Melioidosis as a Cause of Acute Abdomen in Immuno-Competent Male from Eastern India. J Lab Physicians 2015; 7(1): 58–60.

17. Sugi Subramaniam RV, et al. Intra-Abdominal Melioidosis Masquerading as a Tubercular Abdomen: Report of a Rare Case and Literature Review. Surg Infect (Larchmt) 2013; 14(3): 319–21.

18. Tan HJ, et al. Laparoscopic Approach for Pancreato-Splenic Abscess from Disseminated Melioidosis: Surgical Outcome and Review of Literature. J Case Reports 2021; 5: 241.

19. Appukkuttan A, et al. Lesser Sac Haematoma – Meliodosis: A Surgical Surprise. J Evid Based Med 2021; 8: 2349–570.

20. Martin PF, et al. Melioidosis: A Rare Cause of Liver Abscess. Case Reports Hepatol 2016; 2016: 5910375.

21. Vidyalakshmi K, et al. Emerging Clinico-Epidemiological Trends in Melioidosis: Analysis of 95 Cases from Western Coastal India. Int J Infect Dis 2012; 16(7): e491–e7.

22. McRobb E, et al. Melioidosis from Contaminated Bore Water and Successful UV Sterilization. Am J Trop Med Hyg 2013; 89(2): 367–8.

23. Tipre M, et al. Melioidosis in India and Bangladesh: A Review of Case Reports. Asian Pac J Trop Med 2018; 11(5): 320–29.

24. Chang CY. Pyomyositis Masquerading as Suprapubic Mass: An Unusual Presentation of Melioidosis. Ceylon Med J 2021; 66(2): 102–4.

25. Morse LP, et al. Prostatic Abscess Due to *Burkholderia pseudomallei*: 81 Cases from a 19-Year Prospective Melioidosis Study. J Urol 2009; 182(2): 542–7; discussion 47.

26. Currie BJ, et al. Endemic Melioidosis in Tropical Northern Australia: A 10-Year Prospective Study and Review of the Literature. Clin Infect Dis 2000; 31(4): 981–6.

27. Chien JM, et al. Factors Affecting Clinical Outcomes in the Management of Melioidosis in Singapore: A 16-Year Case Series. BMC Infect Dis 2018; 18(1): 482.

28. Kozlowska J, et al. Prostatic Abscess Due to *Burkholderia pseudomallei*: Facilitating Diagnosis to Optimize Management. Am J Trop Med Hyg 2018; 98(1): 227–30.

29. Koshy M, et al. Genitourinary Melioidosis: A Descriptive Study. Trop Doct 2019; 49(2): 104–7.

30. Puthucheary SD, et al. Septicaemic Melioidosis: A Review of 50 Cases from Malaysia. Trans R Soc Trop Med Hyg 1992; 86(6): 683–5.

31. Dhiensiri T, et al. Visceral Abscess in Melioidosis. J Med Assoc Thai 1995; 78(5): 225–31.

32. Chaowagul W, et al. Melioidosis: A Major Cause of Community-Acquired Septicemia in Northeastern Thailand. J Infect Dis 1989; 159(5): 890–9.

33. Punyagupta S. Melioidosis. Review of 686 cases and presentation of a new clinical classification. In: Punyagupta S, Sirisanthana T, Stapatayavong B, eds. Melioidosis. Bangkok, Thailand: Bangkok Medical Publisher; 1989: 217–29.

34. Tan JK, et al. Primary Melioidotic Prostatic Abscess: Presentation, Diagnosis and Management. ANZ J Surg 2002; 72(6): 408–10.

Neuromelioidosis 11

Menka Jha
Department of Neurology, All India Institute of Medical Sciences, Bhubaneswar, India

Suprava Naik
Department of Radiodiagnosis, All India Institute of Medical Sciences, Bhubaneswar, India

Sanjeev Kumar Bhoi
Department of Neurology, All India Institute of Medical Sciences, Bhubaneswar, India

Contents

INTRODUCTION

Burkholderia pseudomallei is a facultative soil saprophyte Gram-negative bacillus, commonly affecting the lungs in the form of pneumonia.[1] Though rare, it can affect the central nervous system (CNS), causing multiple brain abscesses and other manifestations. It belongs to the *Burkholderia* genus. Other pathogenic members in this genus are *B. mallei*, *B. cenocepacia*, etc. *B. mallei* causes glanders in horses and other solipeds

DOI: 10.1201/9781003324010-11

and is highly virulent in humans. *B. cenocepacia* is an essential cause of opportunistic infection in patients with cystic fibrosis.

EPIDEMIOLOGY

It is endemic in tropical regions, which include Southeast Asia, Northern Australia, India, and China. The first report of CNS melioidosis was presented in 1977. Most cases (93%) are reported from the endemic areas of melioidosis, and 7% are from the non-endemic countries like the United States, Belgium, Japan, Norway, and the United Arab Emirates.[2,3] These patients had a history of residence in the endemic areas. Melioidosis is predominantly seasonal; 75–81% of cases occur during the rainy season.

The median age of presentation of CNS melioidosis is 40 years. The youngest case reported was a 10-day-old newborn, while the oldest was 75 years old.[4] Adults are more commonly affected than children (77%) and a male preponderance (70%) is reported in the literature.[4] Melioidosis has been transmitted to infants through breast milk from mothers with mastitis.

Melioidosis can affect many organs, but neurological involvement is rare. Only 1–5% of melioidosis cases have been reported to have neurological affection.[2,3,5] The incidence of CNS involvement in one of the largest case series from India was 1%.[6] In another case series, 32 patients did not report any neurological involvement,[7] though case reports of neuromelioidosis have been reported from various centres.

PATHOGENESIS

Melioidosis primarily affects persons who are in regular contact with soil and water. The pathogenesis appears to be different among the cases. Hematogenous spread to the CNS plays an important role in transmitting the organisms, as evidenced by the highest culture positivity from blood culture specimens. The circulating bacteria can cross the cellular barriers using the transcellular, paracellular, or Trojan horse method.[8] Infection can also result from the percutaneous injection (e.g., through a penetrating injury or open wound), inhalation, or ingestion (e.g., through contaminated food or water). It can enter the brain through the olfactory and trigeminal nerve, bypassing the blood-brain barrier, especially in the encephalomyelitis type.[9]

B. pseudomallei can invade macrophages and may survive and replicate for prolonged periods. After phagocytosis, some bacteria are destroyed, and a proportion of the organisms escape endocytic vacuoles and either break out directly to the extracellular space or infect other cells through actin-based membrane protrusions. Toll-like receptors (TLRs) expressed on host cells are the first to detect invading *B. pseudomallei*, leading to nuclear factor-κB (NF-κB)-induced activation of the immune response through the release of proinflammatory cytokines. Neutrophils are recruited toward the site of infection, and the complement and coagulation cascade become activated. As the infection progresses, the adaptive immune response leads to T-cell recruitment in response to interferon-γ production, which gives rise to a cell-mediated immune response and the production of antibodies by B cells.

RISK FACTORS

Up to 80% of patients with melioidosis have one or more risk factors.[2,6] Risk factors for melioidosis include diabetes (present in 23–60% of patients), heavy alcohol use (in 12–39%), chronic pulmonary disease (in 12–27%), chronic renal disease (in 10–27%), thalassemia (in 7%), glucocorticoid therapy (in <5%), and cancer (in <5%). A previously healthy person is unlikely to have a fatal outcome if the infection is diagnosed early and appropriate antibiotic agents and intensive care resources are available.

CLINICAL FEATURES

It can present as pneumonia, genitourinary infection, skin infection, bacteraemia without evident focus, septic arthritis or osteomyelitis, and neurologic involvement. Severity varies from an acute fulminant septic illness to a chronic infection that may mimic cancer or tuberculosis. Internal-organ abscesses and secondary foci in the lungs, joints, or both are common.

CNS melioidosis is a heterogeneous disease that can present as encephalomyelitis, brain abscess, isolated myelitis, isolated meningitis, or extra-axial collection.[2,4,10,11]

Fever is the most common manifestation, followed by headache, which is seen in the majority of the cases on admission. Focal neurological deficits, especially cranial nerve palsies, are prominent features in the encephalitic form. The common site of affection is mainly the brainstem. Sixth, seven, ninth, and tenth, and more importantly, trigeminal nerve involvement is commonly seen. The differential diagnosis of this form includes *Listeria monocytogenes*, herpes simplex type 1 and mycobacterium tuberculosis.[12–14]

For the brain abscess type, unilateral limb weakness or hemiparesis may be the presenting feature along with fever and headache, though cranial nerve palsy also occurs infrequently. Cerebellar signs can also be seen. Patients with pure myelitis usually present with classic spinal cord syndrome and require a high index of suspicion for the diagnosis.

The initial presentation can also be cranial swelling like scalp abscess, parotid abscess, or orbital abscess.

DIAGNOSIS

Cerebrospinal Fluid Study

The cerebrospinal fluid (CSF) profile of CNS melioidosis includes elevated white cell counts with lymphomononuclear predominance, which commonly mimics tubercular or viral meningitis.[4,15] In one-third, polymorphonuclear cells predominance can be seen, which is also seen in *Listeria meningoencephalitis*. The CSF protein is elevated in the majority, with glucose being slightly elevated to normal. It helps to differentiate between tubercular and fungal aetiology in which glucose is characteristically lower. CSF culture positivity is less as compared to blood culture.

Neuroradiology

A brain CT scan done early in the disease can be normal. Contrast-enhanced magnetic resonance imaging (MRI) is the study of choice as it is abnormal in almost all cases of melioidosis with neurological involvement. CNS melioidosis in MRI commonly appears as a rounded or tubular rim enhancing microabscesses.[15] Other CNS infections that may resemble melioidosis micro-abscesses include toxoplasmosis, neurocysticercosis, and tuberculosis. It shows the tendency to involve and spread along white-matter tracts across the commissural and projection fibres to the contralateral hemisphere.[15,16] The white-matter tracts involved include the corpus callosum, corticospinal tracts, trigeminal nuclei, and cerebellar peduncles. Another characteristic of the micro-abscesses is restricted diffusion on DWI (diffusion weighted imaging) and corresponding low signal on ADC (apparent diffusion coefficient) maps (Figure 11.1). Rarely, features of skull osteomyelitis, extradural abscess, and leptomeningeal thickening can be seen adjacent to the parenchymal lesion. This invasive behaviour is similar to tuberculosis, invasive fungal infection, and malignant neoplasm.

Cranial nerve involvement can be seen as the thickening and enhancement of the cisternal segment of the nerve tracking to its brainstem nucleus. This peculiar imaging feature may give a clue on the perineural route of entry of *B. pseudomallei* into the CNS. Other neurotropic infections, such as members of herpes viridae, *Borrelia burgdorferi,* and *Listeria monocytogenes* can also involve the cranial nerves, usually manifesting as cranial nerve thickening and enhancement.[17–19] The distinguishing feature of CNS melioidosis is that cranial nerve disease is much more extensive and shows contiguous intra-axial spread into the brain stem, resulting in micro-abscesses (Figures 11.1 and 11.2).

Culture

Culture from the CNS specimen is the gold standard for the diagnosis of CNS melioidosis.[20] The sources can include brain tissue, pus from the abscess or subdural

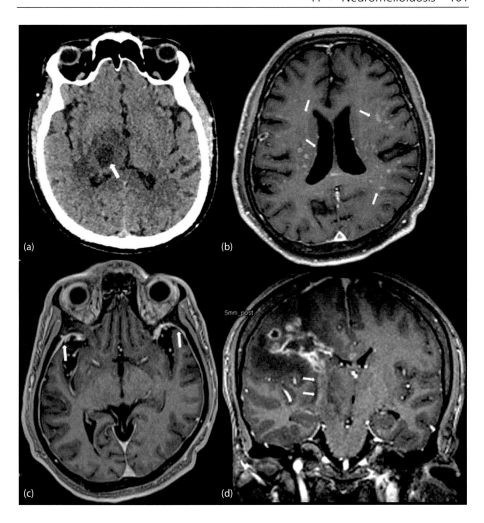

FIGURE 11.1 Non-contrast CT brain showing hypodense lesion in the right thalamo-capsular area (a). An axial post-contrast T1W MRI of the brain in a 35-year-old male melioidosis patient (b and c) shows multiple small nodular and ring-enhancing lesions in the bilateral cerebral hemisphere (arrows in b) and pachymeningeal enhancement (arrows in c). Coronal post-contrast T1WI (d) in another patient shows multiple small abscesses, some coalesced centrally and extending along the corticospinal tract and the corpus callosum (arrows in d).

collection, and CSF. Tissue from the brainstem can be difficult to obtain, so in suspected CNS disease, positive culture from other sites helps in diagnosis. Blood culture has the highest sensitivity (52%), others being sputum, pus from skin lesion, splenic pus, skull osteomyelitis, or scalp abscess. Though serology and polymerase chain reaction positivity have been reported; they are unreliable.

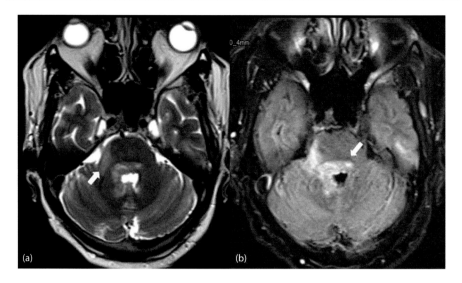

FIGURE 11.2   Axial T2W (a) and FLAIR (b) MRI of the brain of a 36-year-old melioidosis patient shows hyperintensity in the region of the right trigeminal nerve nucleus and dorsal pons.

TREATMENT

CNS melioidosis is treatment-resistant and requires long-term management. Treatment consists of two phases; the first intensive phase, for 8 weeks, consists of parenteral antibiotics in which ceftazidime and meropenem are the drugs of choice. Other drugs like doxycycline and chloramphenicol have also been used with a very low success rate. In the second 6-month maintenance phase, trimethoprim/sulfamethoxazole (TMP/SMX) is used as the first-line drug. However, doxycycline and amoxycillin/clavulanic acid have also been used in patients who cannot tolerate TMP/SMX. The treatment duration is also important, which consists of at least 8 weeks for the intensive phase and 6 months or longer for the eradication phase.[21] Where feasible, adjunctive surgical procedures like abscess drainage may be required in addition to the antibiotics.

If treated early in the course and for an adequate duration, most cases recover completely or partially with some neurological sequelae, like residual paresis, facial weakness, or ataxia (Figure 11.3). Overall mortality reported in various case series is 20%, though it can range from 21% to 50%, which is significantly higher than the non-neurological case.[2,10,15] Recurrent melioidosis can occur if treatment adherence is poor.

As melioidosis can mimic various infectious diseases, it should be considered in the differential diagnosis of meningoencephalitis and intracranial abscess with poor treatment response and rapid clinical progression. Timely initiation of sensitive antibiotics for an adequate duration is the key to successful treatment and preventing fatal outcomes and significant neurological sequelae.

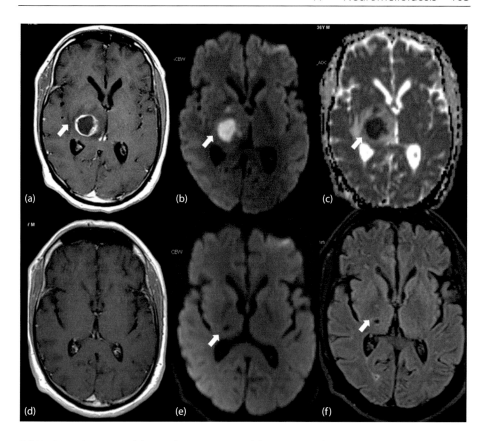

FIGURE 11.3 A cranial MRI in a 36-year-old patient with neuromelioidosis shows a peripherally enhancing lesion in the right thalamus (a). The lesion shows central diffusion restriction on the diffusion-weighted image (b) with ADC reversal (c). Follow-up imaging after 1 year of treatment shows resolution of the abscess (d, e, and f).

REFERENCES

1. Wiersinga WJ, et al. Melioidosis: Insights into the Pathogenicity of *Burkholderia pseudomallei*. Nat Rev Microbiol 2006; 4(4): 272–82.
2. Currie BJ, et al. The Epidemiology and Clinical spectrum of Melioidosis: 540 Cases from the 20 Year Darwin Prospective Study. PLoS Negl Trop Dis 2010; 4(11): e900.
3. Limmathurotsakul D, et al. Variable Presentation of Neurological Melioidosis in Northeast Thailand. Am J Trop Med Hyg 2007; 77(1): 118–20.
4. Wongwandee M, et al. Central Nervous System Melioidosis: A Systematic Review of Individual Participant Data of Case Reports and Case Series. PLoS Negl Trop Dis 2019; 13(4): e0007320.
5. Vidyalakshmi K, et al. Emerging Clinico-Epidemiological Trends in Melioidosis: Analysis of 95 Cases from Western Coastal India. Int J Infect Dis 2012; 16(7): e491–7.

6. Hassan MR, et al. Incidence, Risk Factors and Clinical Epidemiology of Melioidosis: A Complex Socio-Ecological Emerging Infectious Disease in the Alor Setar Region of Kedah, Malaysia. BMC Infect Dis 2010; 10: 302.

7. Gopalakrishnan R, et al. Melioidosis: An Emerging Infection in India. J Assoc Physicians India 2013; 61(9): 612–4.

8. St John JA. Trojan Horse L-Selectin Monocytes: A Portal of *Burkholderia pseudomallei* Entry into the Brain. Virulence 2017; 8(6): 611–2.

9. St John JA, et al. *Burkholderia pseudomallei* Rapidly Infects the Brain Stem and Spinal Cord via the Trigeminal Nerve after Intranasal Inoculation. Infect Immun 2016; 84(9): 2681–8.

10. Deuble M, et al. Neurologic Melioidosis. Am J Trop Med Hyg 2013; 89(3): 535–9.

11. Kumar GS, et al. Cranial Melioidosis Presenting as a Mass Lesion or Osteomyelitis. J Neurosurg 2008; 108(2): 243–7.

12. Mylonakis E, et al. Central Nervous System Infection with Listeria Monocytogenes. 33 years' Experience at a General Hospital and Review of 776 Episodes from the Literature. Medicine (Baltimore) 1998; 77(5): 313–36.

13. Whitley RJ, et al. Diseases That Mimic Herpes Simplex Encephalitis. Diagnosis, Presentation, and Outcome. NIAD Collaborative Antiviral Study Group. JAMA 1989; 262(2): 234–9.

14. Kennedy DH, et al. Tuberculous Meningitis. JAMA 1979; 241(3): 264–8.

15. Currie BJ, et al. Neurological Melioidosis. Acta Trop 2000; 74(2-3): 145–51.

16. Hsu CC, et al. Neuromelioidosis: Craniospinal MRI Findings in *Burkholderia pseudomallei* Infection. J Neuroimaging 2016; 26(1): 75–82.

17. Hildenbrand P, et al. Lyme Neuroborreliosis: Manifestations of a Rapidly Emerging Zoonosis. AJNR Am J Neuroradiol 2009; 30(6): 1079–87.

18. Moro A, et al. Rhombencephalitis Caused by Listeria Monocytogenes with Striking Involvement of Trigeminal Nerve on MR Imaging. Arq Neuropsiquiatr 2011; 69(3): 568–9.

19. Tien RD, et al. Herpes Trigeminal Neuritis and Rhombencephalitis on Gd-DTPA-Enhanced MR Imaging. AJNR Am J Neuroradiol 1990; 11(2): 413–4.

20. Wiersinga WJ, et al. Melioidosis. N Engl J Med 2012; 367(11): 1035–44.

21. Lipsitz R, et al. Workshop on Treatment of and Postexposure Prophylaxis for *Burkholderia pseudomallei* and *B. mallei* Infection, 2010. Emerg Infect Dis 2012; 18(12): e2.

Gastrointestinal Melioidosis

12

Abhijeet Rai

Department of Gastroenterology, All India Institute of Medical Sciences, Bhubaneswar, India

Hemanta K Nayak

Department of Gastroenterology, All India Institute of Medical Sciences, Bhubaneswar, India

Manas K Panigrahi

Department of Gastroenterology, All India Institute of Medical Sciences, Bhubaneswar, India

Contents

DOI: 10.1201/9781003324010-12

INTRODUCTION

Melioidosis, also known as Whitmore's disease, is an infectious disease caused by the bacterium *Burkholderia pseudomallei*, whose natural habitat includes soil and fresh-water source in tropical and subtropical regions of the world.[1] The disease prevalence is highly under-recognized and under-reported because of a lack of awareness among clinicians and a lack of laboratory facilities. There is a wide range of manifestations of melioidosis, making clinical diagnosis often challenging. Furthermore, melioidosis is a close mimicker of tuberculosis, which is highly endemic in India. Many patients receive antitubercular therapy, which delays its diagnosis and substantially increases morbidity and mortality.[2]

The bacterium usually enters the body through the skin or inhalation route. People living in rural areas and involved in agriculture work are more predisposed to acquire the organism while working in fields or in freshwater sources. There have been many case reports and case series published from India on gastrointestinal melioidosis. It is gradually recognized as a fatal disease in India and the neighbouring Southeast Asia region.

RISK FACTORS

The most important and common risk factor for gastrointestinal melioidosis is diabetes mellitus, which accounts for more than half of the patients.[3] Other risk factors include male gender, exposure to soil and freshwater sources, and chronic comorbid illness such as chronic liver disease, chronic kidney disease, prolonged immunosuppression, and primary and secondary iron overload state.[4] However, in up to one-fifth of cases, no definite risk factors were identified.[5] Zoonotic transmission is also uncommon.

PATHOPHYSIOLOGY

B. pseudomallei is a facultative intracellular bacterium with multiple virulence factors that play a crucial role in the pathogenesis of the disease. Capsular polysaccharides and type IV pilin play an important role in host-cell adhesion and invasion.[6] Host factors also play a role in cellular invasion, as demonstrated by cells having protease-activated receptor 1 being susceptible to cellular adhesion, invasion, growth, and dissemination.[7]

B. pseudomallei resists intracellular degradation by suppressing intracellular nitric oxide synthase (iNOS).[8] Further intercellular spread of bacteria results in fusion of cells and the formation of multi-nuclear giant cells, a hallmark of melioidosis.[9] Lysis of these giant cells results in the formation of plaques, which act as a nidus for latent or persistent infection.[10]

CLINICAL FEATURES

Most *B. pseudomallei* infections are usually asymptomatic.[11] However, patients with underlying chronic comorbid illness and immunosuppression are predisposed to developing severe illness. The normal incubation period ranges from 1 day to 3 weeks with an average of 9 days;[12] however, it may be shorter when the infection is acquired by inhalation or aspiration of contaminated freshwater.[13] It may manifest clinically as acute, subacute, or chronic infection, with acute infection being the most common presentation.[14]

Acute Infection

Gastrointestinal melioidosis mainly presents as community-acquired pneumonia but can also involve the skin and genitourinary tract. More than 50% of patients with acute infections have bacteraemia. One-quarter of patients may have septic shock at presentation, with the mortality rate of acute infection ranging from 10% to 40%.[5]

Chronic Infection

Patients with chronic melioidosis are usually symptomatic for a few months and primarily present with chronic pulmonary symptoms mimicking tuberculosis, non-healing skin ulcers, or abscesses.[14] Chronic infection has a significantly lower mortality rate of 2% compared to acute infection.[14]

Latent Infection with Recrudescence

On rare occasions, infection with *B. pseudomallei* can have a prolonged latent phase and may relapse later in life. However, this phenomenon is relatively uncommon.[14] Large retrospective studies have shown that the most common presentation is pneumonia, followed by genitourinary infection, skin infection, bacteraemia, septic arthritis, and neurologic involvement, and rarely involves the gastrointestinal system.[14]

GASTROINTESTINAL INVOLVEMENT IN MELIOIDOSIS

Melioidosis can have diverse manifestations in the gastrointestinal system. Many case reports and case series have described melioidosis as a rare cause of liver and splenic abscess. Late pancreatic melioidosis has also been reported as a pancreatic abscess or infected pseudocyst.[15]

Oesophageal Melioidosis

Primary involvement of the oesophagus by melioidosis is not reported in the literature. However, few case reports have shown the involvement of the oesophagus secondary to bronchial tree involvement and usually presented with dysphagia, loss of weight, and appetite. Such unusual presentation poses a diagnostic challenge and may present as a non-healing oesophago-bronchial fistula, requiring an exhaustive workup and multi-disciplinary management. It is more challenging for the closure of the fistula between the left main bronchus and oesophagus. A multi-disciplinary team approach with endoscopic covered metallic stenting is required for closure of fistula in addition to long-term antibiotics therapy. The possibility of melioidosis may be considered in a patient with broncho-oesophageal fistula with lung consolidation and septicaemia in the background of diabetes in endemic areas.

Hepatic Melioidosis

Isolated liver abscess is extremely rare, and its involvement is limited to disseminated cases. Liver abscess by melioidosis is clinically indistinguishable from other causes of pyogenic liver abscess and tubercular abscess. It usually presents with prolonged high-grade fever, not responding to usual empiric antibiotics, and occasionally may present with right upper-quadrant pain and jaundice.[16–18] Many case series have described CT findings in hepatic melioidosis as 'honeycomb pattern' and 'necklace sign' of multi-septated multi-loculated lesions (Figure 12.1).[19] CT scan findings of peripheral enhancement with a 'honeycomb' appearance increase the suspicion, especially in the presence of other affected intra-abdominal organs such as the spleen.[3,4] A definitive diagnosis

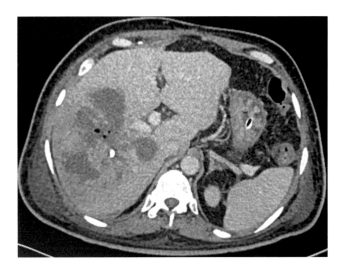

FIGURE 12.1   A CT scan of an abdomen showing 'honeycomb sign' with asymmetric locules of varying sizes, characteristic of melioidosis.

was established by Gram staining and culture studies. Melioidosis liver abscesses often require percutaneous drainage and sometimes surgical drainage as these patients are often critically ill.

Biliary Melioidosis

The gallbladder and biliary tract are rarely involved in melioidosis. However, the exact reason is unknown, but probably due to a relative lack of blood supply as compared to other common sites of involvement like the lung and musculoskeletal system. Few case reports have been described in the literature where melioidosis presents as acute acalculous cholecystitis or cholangitis.[20] There is often delayed diagnostic because of rarity. Treatment requires early cholecystectomy followed by prolonged broad-spectrum antibiotic therapy. Cholangitis usually requires urgent endoscopic biliary drainage.

Splenic Melioidosis

The spleen is the most commonly involved abdominal organ, followed by the liver, in gastrointestinal melioidosis.[21] It generally presents as hepatosplenic abscesses, and involvement of both the liver and spleen may give a clue to the diagnosis of melioidosis.[21] The involvement of the spleen can occur either as a manifestation of both acute and chronic infection. The acute phase is generally a part of multi-organ involvement, with other organ manifestations dominating the clinical picture. The chronic form often presents as isolated splenic involvement and is usually asymptomatic.[21] However, there are rare reports of the chronic phase of involvement presenting as ruptured splenic abscess and peritonitis.[22] Occasionally, multiple peripherally distributed abscesses may give to a contained rupture without any signs of peritonitis.[23] Imaging findings are, although not-specific, commonly present as single or multiple splenic abscesses (Figure 12.2). Tuberculosis, brucellosis, and fungal infection are differential diagnoses of such clinical and imaging features. Early diagnosis and aggressive treatment with surgical drainage and antibiotics decrease mortality and morbidity for several weeks.

Pancreatic Melioidosis

Pancreatic involvement of melioidosis is rarely reported, with only a handful of cases published until now, and usually presents as a bulky pancreas with large focal abscesses or multiple micro-abscesses.[14] Associated peripancreatic fat stranding and splenic vein thrombosis can be seen. However, amylase lipase levels are generally normal despite abscess formation in the pancreas.[14] In rare cases, only changes of acute interstitial pancreatitis without pancreatic abscess can be seen.[23] Recently, reports of melioidosis-infected pancreatic pseudocyst were reported in the literature with good outcomes following endoscopic ultrasound (EUS) guided cystogastrostomy and prolonged antibiotics (Figures 12.3 and 12.4).[24]

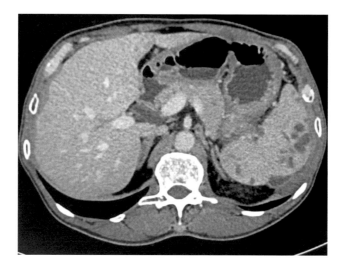

FIGURE 12.2   A CT scan showing multiple peripherally distributed abscesses in the spleen, suggestive of isolated splenic melioidosis (chronic phase).

Intestinal Melioidosis

Scant literature is available about intestinal involvement with melioidosis and its clinical manifestations. A case was reported from the Indian subcontinent, where intestinal melioidosis presented as an acute abdomen with perforation peritonitis. He underwent exploratory laparotomy, which showed two ileal perforations with

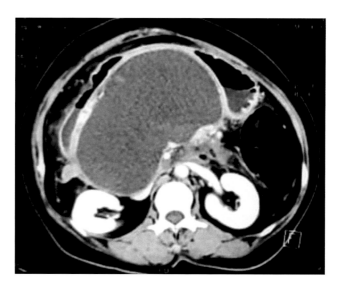

FIGURE 12.3   A CT scan showing a large pancreatic pseudocyst abutting the gastric wall.

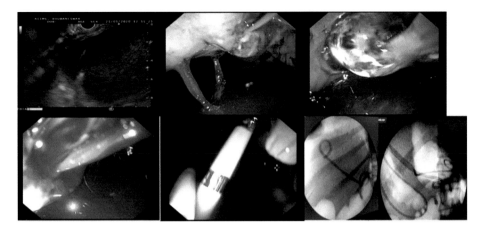

FIGURE 12.4   Steps of EUS-guided cystogastrostomy, from left to right: EUS visualization of the pseudocyst, passing cystotome followed by guidewire through the gastric wall into pseudocyst, balloon dilation of the tract, placement of double pigtail stent in the cyst cavity with one end in the gastric lumen, and fluoroscopic image for confirming the position of the stent.

intra-abdominal purulent fluid, which grows *B. pseudomallei*,[25] successfully managed with omental patch closure of the perforation and pelvic drain placement and long-term antibiotics.

MICROBIOLOGICAL DIAGNOSIS

Culture

As mentioned earlier, *B. pseudomallei* can be grown on routine culture media. Still, because of a lack of clinical suspicion by treating physicians and the unfamiliarity of laboratory personnel with the colony characteristics, microbial growth could be neglected and attributed to environmental contamination.[26] *B. pseudomallei* is not a part of normal human flora, and its detection in any clinical sample is diagnostic of melioidosis. Sending properly collected samples such as pus is of utmost importance in diagnosing melioidosis. Blood culture is the most important sample, as bacteraemia is found in most cases. Throat swabs, rectal swabs, and quantitative urine cultures must be sent for all cases of suspected melioidosis.[27,28] The sensitivity of cultures is about 60%, and if the index of suspicion is high, cultures should be repeated as subsequent cultures often are positive.[29] As the bacterium has a slow growth rate and recognizing representative colonies is difficult; it is recommended to use multiple standard biochemical tests and kit-based identification methods to avoid misidentification.[26] Monoclonal antibody-based latex agglutination assay using antigen-antibody binding approach and matrix-assisted laser desorption/ionization time-of-flight (MALDI-TOF) are often used by laboratories to identify *B. pseudomallei* accurately.[30] In a resource-limited setup, it is recommended to use disc diffusion antibiotic sensitivity testing using gentamicin, colistin, and amoxicillin-clavulanic acid to screen all gram-negative isolates that produce cytochrome oxidase,[31] as it might give a clue in the diagnosis of *B. pseudomallei* because of the characteristic antibiotic sensitivity pattern.

Direct Detection in Clinical Samples

As melioidosis can have a fulminant presentation, waiting for cultures before starting treatment is not pragmatic, and detecting the bacterium in clinical samples would expedite clinical decision-making. The textbook definition of the light microscopic appearance of *B. pseudomallei* as a safety pin lacks sensitivity and specificity.[32] Immunofluorescence in microscopy increases the specificity to 100% but still has a sensitivity of only 50% compared to culture.[33] Lateral flow assays using capsular polysaccharide and polymerase chain reaction-based assays using T3 SS gene cluster have been developed, but because of poor sensitivity and high costs involved, they are not used in routine practice.[34,35]

Serology

Many serological assays are available for diagnosing *B. pseudomallei*, but none are widely used because of a lack of standardization. Because of the high background positivity rate in endemic areas, there is a high false-positive rate of such assays.[36] Newer assays are being developed using purified antigens of *B. pseudomallei,* which generates an antibody pattern specific to *B. pseudomallei*, which can improve the serodiagnosis in clinical settings with improved sensitivity and specificity.[37]

TREATMENT

Gastrointestinal melioidosis requires a prolonged course of antibiotics and drainage of abscesses, and source control.

Antibiotic Resistance

B. pseudomallei are intrinsically resistant to penicillin, ampicillin, first- and second-generation cephalosporins, gentamicin, tobramycin, and streptomycin.[38] Antibiotics that are effective against *B. pseudomallei* include beta-lactams like ceftazidime, carbapenems, trimethoprim-sulfamethoxazole (TMP-SMX), and doxycycline.

Intensive Antibiotic Therapy

Intensive therapy is aimed to slow the phase of severe illness in the hospitalized patient. At least 2 weeks of intravenous antibiotic therapy is recommended, followed by long-term oral antibiotics for eradication.[39]

Non-critically ill patients: Ceftazidime 50 mg/kg up to 2 g IV every 6 to 8 hours is generally recommended.[40] Continuous infusion can be given in patients who require early discharge for home IV antibiotic treatment and is pharmacokinetically superior to intermittent dosing.[40]

Critically ill patients: For patients having severe illness requiring ICU care, meropenem (25 mg/kg up to 1 g IV every 8 hours is given as initial therapy. For critically ill patients, the use of meropenem has shown a mortality benefit.[41]

With CNS involvement: In patients with neurological melioidosis, meropenem at a higher dose of 50 mg/kg up to 2 g every 8 hours is recommended, as these patients are often critically ill and have a poor prognosis unless aggressively managed.

Eradication Therapy

Eradication therapy, which begins after the intensive phase, is aimed to prevent the recurrence of melioidosis. Studies have shown that eradication regimes of 12–16 weeks of oral antibiotic therapy have a 90% lower relapse rate than those of 8 weeks of oral antibiotic therapy.[42]

Oral TMP-SMX is preferred for long-term eradication therapy according to weight-based dosing.[43] For a patient who does not tolerate TMP-SMX, doxycycline is an alternative. At least 3 months of eradication therapy is recommended.

PROGNOSIS

Acute melioidosis has a mortality rate of 20–50% worldwide, with higher mortality rates seen in resource-poor countries and people with multiple comorbidities.[44] Risk factors for mortality and treatment failure include bacteraemia, advanced age, and the presence of organ failure.[44] Gastrointestinal melioidosis has an overall good prognosis compared to neurological melioidosis.[45]

CONCLUSION

Gastrointestinal melioidosis may have diverse manifestations. It may present as a rare cause of liver and splenic abscesses. Similarly, pancreatic and peripancreatic inflammation with abscess formation can manifest in pancreatic melioidosis. It is important for clinicians working in both endemic and non-endemic areas to be aware of this rare diagnosis and consider this entity a differential diagnosis.

REFERENCES

1. Limmathurotsakul D, et al. Predicted Global Distribution of *Burkholderia pseudomallei* and Burden of Melioidosis. Nat Microbiol 2016; 1(1): 15008.
2. Mukhopadhyay C, et al. Pediatric Melioidosis in Southern India. Indian Pediatr 2015; 52(8): 711–2.
3. Limmathurotsakul D, et al. Increasing Incidence of Human Melioidosis in Northeast Thailand. Am J Trop Med Hyg 2010; 82(6): 1113–7.
4. Fong SM, et al. Thalassemia Major Is a Major Risk Factor for Pediatric Melioidosis in Kota Kinabalu, Sabah, Malaysia. Clin Infect Dis 2015; 60(12): 1802–7.
5. Currie BJ, et al. Melioidosis Epidemiology and Risk Factors from a Prospective Whole-Population Study in Northern Australia. Trop Med Int Health 2004; 9(11): 1167–74.
6. Essex-Lopresti AE, et al. A Type IV Pilin, Pila, Contributes to Adherence of *Burkholderia pseudomallei* and Virulence in Vivo. Infect Immun 2005; 73(2): 1260–4.
7. Kager LM, et al. Deficiency of Protease-Activated Receptor-1 Limits Bacterial Dissemination During Severe Gram-Negative Sepsis (melioidosis). Microbes Infect 2014; 16(2): 171–4.
8. Ekchariyawat P, et al. *Burkholderia pseudomallei*-Induced Expression of Suppressor of Cytokine Signaling 3 and Cytokine-Inducible Src Homology 2-Containing Protein in Mouse Macrophages: A Possible Mechanism for Suppression of the Response to gamma Interferon Stimulation. Infect Immun 2005; 73(11): 7332–9.
9. Lazar Adler NR, et al. The Molecular and Cellular Basis of Pathogenesis in Melioidosis: How Does *Burkholderia pseudomallei* Cause Disease? FEMS Microbiol Rev 2009; 33(6): 1079–99.
10. French CT, et al. Dissection of the *Burkholderia* Intracellular Life Cycle Using a Photothermal Nanoblade. Proc Natl Acad Sci U S A 2011; 108(29): 12095–100.
11. Cheng AC, et al. Intensity of Exposure and Incidence of Melioidosis in Thai Children. Trans R Soc Trop Med Hyg 2008; 102 Suppl 1: S37–9.
12. Currie BJ, et al. Melioidosis: Acute and Chronic Disease, Relapse and Re-Activation. Trans R Soc Trop Med Hyg 2000; 94(3): 301–4.
13. Chierakul W, et al. Melioidosis in 6 Tsunami Survivors in Southern Thailand. Clin Infect Dis 2005; 41(7): 982–90.
14. Currie BJ, et al. The Darwin Prospective Melioidosis Study: A 30-Year Prospective, Observational Investigation. Lancet Infect Dis 2021; 21(12):1737–46.
15. Chong VH, et al. Pancreatic Involvement in Melioidosis. Jop 2010; 11(4): 365–68.
16. Terrier F, et al. Morphologic Aspects of Hepatic Abscesses at Computed Tomography and Ultrasound. Acta Radiol Diagn (Stockh) 1983; 24(2): 129–37.
17. Wiersinga WJ, et al. Melioidosis. N Engl J Med 2012; 367(11): 1035–44.
18. Vandana KE, et al. Seroprevalence of *Burkholderia pseudomallei* Among Adults in Coastal Areas in Southwestern India. PLoS Negl Trop Dis 2016; 10(4): e0004610.
19. Apisarnthananarak P, et al. Computed Tomography Characteristics of *Burkholderia pseudomallei* Associated Liver Abscess. Clin Infect Dis 2006; 43(12): 1618–20.
20. Mohamad N, et al. Melioidosis in Acute Cholangitis of Diabetic Patient: A Forgotten Diagnosis. Res Rep Trop Med 2012; 3: 103–6.

21. Lim KS, et al. Radiological Manifestations of Melioidosis. Clin Radiol 2010; 65(1): 66–72.

22. Miraclin AT, et al. Septicemic Melioidosis with Ruptured Splenic Abscess in a Patient with Thalassemia Intermedia. J Glob Infect Dis 2017; 9(1): 32–33.

23. Mohan VK, et al. Unusual Presentations of Abdominal Melioidosis. J Glob Infect Dis 2021; 13(1): 52–55.

24. Mahapatra A, et al. Melioidosis in Pancreatic Pseudocyst: Atypical Infection at Atypical Site. Pancreatology 2021; 21(5): 1014–6.

25. Karuna T, et al. Melioidosis as a Cause of Acute Abdomen in Immuno-Competent Male from Eastern India. J Lab Physicians 2015; 7(1): 58–60.

26. Hoffmaster AR, et al. Melioidosis Diagnostic Workshop, 2013. Emerg Infect Dis 2015; 21(2): e141045.

27. Wuthiekanun V, et al. Value of Throat Swab in Diagnosis of Melioidosis. J Clin Microbiol 2001; 39(10): 3801–2.

28. Limmathurotsakul D, et al. Role and Significance of Quantitative Urine Cultures in Diagnosis of Melioidosis. J Clin Microbiol 2005; 43(5): 2274–6.

29. Limmathurotsakul D, et al. Defining the True Sensitivity of Culture for the Diagnosis of Melioidosis Using Bayesian Latent Class Models. PLoS One 2010; 5(8): e12485.

30. Suttisunhakul V, et al. Matrix-Assisted Laser desorption/ionization Time-of-Flight Mass Spectrometry for the Identification of *Burkholderia pseudomallei* from Asia and Australia and Differentiation between *Burkholderia* Species. PLoS One 2017; 12(4): e0175294.

31. Dance DA, et al. *Burkholderia pseudomallei:* Challenges for the Clinical Microbiology Laboratory-a Response from the Front Line. J Clin Microbiol 2017; 55(3): 980–82.

32. Sheridan EA, et al. Evaluation of the Wayson Stain for the Rapid Diagnosis of Melioidosis. J Clin Microbiol 2007; 45(5): 1669–70.

33. Tandhavanant S, et al. Monoclonal Antibody-Based Immunofluorescence Microscopy for the Rapid Identification of *Burkholderia pseudomallei* in Clinical Specimens. Am J Trop Med Hyg 2013; 89(1): 165–8.

34. Houghton RL, et al. Development of a Prototype Lateral Flow Immunoassay (LFI) for the Rapid Diagnosis of Melioidosis. PLoS Negl Trop Dis 2014; 8(3): e2727.

35. Kaestli M, et al. Comparison of TaqMan PCR Assays for Detection of the Melioidosis Agent *Burkholderia pseudomallei* in Clinical Specimens. J Clin Microbiol 2012; 50(6): 2059–62.

36. Cheng AC, et al. Prospective Evaluation of a Rapid Immunochromogenic Cassette Test for the Diagnosis of Melioidosis in Northeast Thailand. Trans R Soc Trop Med Hyg 2006; 100(1): 64–7.

37. Kohler C, et al. Rapid and Sensitive Multiplex Detection of *Burkholderia pseudomallei-* Specific Antibodies in Melioidosis Patients Based on a Protein Microarray Approach. PLoS Negl Trop Dis 2016; 10(7): e0004847.

38. Leelarasamee A, et al. Melioidosis: Review and Update. Rev Infect Dis 1989; 11(3): 413–25.

39. White NJ, et al. Halving of Mortality of Severe Melioidosis by Ceftazidime. Lancet 1989; 2(8665): 697–701.

40. Angus BJ, et al. Pharmacokinetic-Pharmacodynamic Evaluation of Ceftazidime Continuous Infusion vs. Intermittent Bolus Injection in Septicaemic Melioidosis. Br J Clin Pharmacol 2000; 50(2): 184–91.

41. Stephens DP, et al. Melioidosis Causing Critical Illness: A Review of 24 Years of Experience from the Royal Darwin Hospital ICU. Crit Care Med 2016; 44(8): 1500–5.

42. Limmathurotsakul D, et al. Risk Factors for Recurrent Melioidosis in Northeast Thailand. Clin Infect Dis 2006; 43(8): 979–86.

43. Chetchotisakd P, et al. Trimethoprim-Sulfamethoxazole Versus Trimethoprim-Sulfamethoxazole Plus Doxycycline as Oral Eradicative Treatment for Melioidosis (MERTH): A Multicentre, Double-Blind, non-Inferiority, Randomised Controlled Trial. Lancet 2014; 383(9919): 807–14.
44. Chierakul W, et al. Two Randomized Controlled Trials of Ceftazidime Alone Versus Ceftazidime in Combination with Trimethoprim-Sulfamethoxazole for the Treatment of Severe Melioidosis. Clin Infect Dis 2005; 41(8): 1105–13.
45. Currie BJ, et al. Neurological Melioidosis. Acta Trop 2000; 74(2-3): 145–51.

Septicaemic Melioidosis

13

Prasanta R Mohapatra

Department of Pulmonary Medicine and Critical Care,
All India Institute of Medical Sciences, Bhubaneswar, India

Ananda Datta

Department of Pulmonary Medicine and Critical Care,
All India Institute of Medical Sciences, Bhubaneswar, India

Contents

Sepsis of any aetiology is a life-threatening condition requiring urgent and effective antimicrobial therapy. Identifying the site of infection, the potential pathogens, and the judicious use of antibiotics is a priority. Sepsis can be community-acquired, and evolution can be aggressive, confirming that the cause is complex.[1,2] The outcome depends on control of many determinants, early use of appropriate antibiotics, and effective source control.[3]

Melioidosis is caused by the Gram-negative aerobic bacterium *Burkholderia pseudomallei*. Septicaemic melioidosis accounts for nearly 25% (66/255) of community-acquired bacteremia in Northeast Thailand[4] and is the most common cause of fatal

DOI: 10.1201/9781003324010-13

community-acquired bacteremic pneumonia in tropical northern Australia and north-east Thailand.[5,6]

In the intensive care unit (ICU), sepsis has been the common cause of death. The causative microorganism often remains unidentified; particularly, it is difficult to find an uncommon aetiology, like melioidosis. These patients had a high predilection for multiple comorbidities and underlying diseases in this setting.[6,7] Recent case series from Malaysia have shown that the common clinical presentation of acute melioidosis was pneumonia (61.6%), internal organ abscesses (49.3%), and localized soft-tissue infection (21.9%). The blood culture was positive only in 64.4% of cases. Pneumonia, along with bacteremia, was associated with sepsis and septic shock. But the patients having soft-tissue infections or abscesses generally had a milder form of melioidosis. Abnormal blood parameters like renal function tests (serum urea, creatinine, serum bicarbonate, etc.) and liver function tests (protein, albumin, and aspartate transaminase) were associated with increased mortality on univariate analysis (all P <0.05). On multi-variate analysis, low serum bicarbonate (P = 0.004, OR 0.64, 95% CI 0.48–0.87) and albumin (P = 0.031, OR 0.73, 95% CI 0.54–0.97) had been associated with higher mortality.[8]

There have been continuous advancements in the understanding of the pathophysiology and mechanism of the development of sepsis, which is considered a dysregulated host reaction to the infection involving not only the activation of the pro- and anti-inflammatory responses but also alterations in cardiovascular, autonomic, neurological, hormonal, metabolic, and clotting pathways.

SEPSIS IN GENERAL

Sepsis and septic shock are major threats to the global healthcare system, affecting millions annually. It is not only associated with a mortality rate of 42% but also can lead to long-term physical and mental morbidity and disability. It is a time-sensitive medical emergency. Early detection and prompt institution of appropriate management can improve outcomes.[9] According to the *Third International Consensus Definitions for Sepsis and Septic Shock* (Sepsis-3),[10] sepsis is defined as 'life-threatening organ dysfunction caused by a dysregulated host response to infection'. Septic shock is a subset of sepsis in which underlying circulatory and cellular/metabolic abnormalities are profound enough to increase mortality substantially. For clinical operationalization, organ dysfunction can be represented by an increase in the sequential organ failure assessment (SOFA) score of two points or more from baseline, associated with in-hospital mortality more significantly than 10%. SOFA is a standard system that uses available parameters in routine hospital practice to identify the dysfunction or failure of the key organs due to sepsis. Despite the individual variation and subjectivity, the SOFA score appropriately correlated to the further evolution of the patient. Irrespective of the initial SOFA score, an increase in subsequent scores during the initial 48 hours in the ICU predicts a mortality rate of at least 50%.[11] Patients with septic shock can be clinically identified by the requirement of vasopressor to maintain a mean arterial pressure of 65 mm Hg or greater in case of persistent hypotension, and the patients who have serum lactate levels greater than 2 mmol/L (>18 mg/dL) in the absence of hypovolemia. These criteria indicate hospital mortality rates greater than 40%. In out-of-hospital, emergency department, or general hospital ward settings, adult patients with suspected infection can be rapidly identified using a bedside clinical score known as quick SOFA (qSOFA) that consists of three clinical criteria: A respiratory rate of 22/min or greater, altered mentation, and systolic blood pressure of 100 mm Hg or less. A score of at least two denotes poor outcomes in patients with suspected infection and prompts clinicians to initiate a more elaborated search for organ dysfunction.[10] However, the *Surviving Sepsis Campaign* guidelines recommended against using qSOFA as a single screening stool for sepsis and septic shock.[9]

Tissue perfusion at the regional level may be compromised often before the development of overt hypotension.[13] Serum lactate is a surrogate marker for this tissue hypoperfusion.[12] Moreover, tissue perfusion may remain impaired even after aggressive resuscitation due to microcirculatory failure.[13] Being a virulent bacteria, infection with *B. pseudomallei* can progress to sepsis and septic shock.[14] The case fatality rate depends on the extent of delay in antibiotic therapy; it can be as high as 90% without treatment. Early intensive care and empirical administration of appropriate antibiotics can reduce mortality substantially.

CLINICAL PRESENTATION

The incubation period of acute septicaemic melioidosis is the shortest. The average incubation period of acute melioidosis is nine days. But it may vary from 1 to 21 days. Generally, acute presentation has been described as symptoms lasting less than 2 months.[15] This type is very common and presents as fulminant community-acquired pneumonia and sepsis with high mortality. Its clinical manifestation is dependent on the involvement of different organs. It is worth mentioning that the clinical spectrum of melioidosis varies from symptomatic acute presentation to asymptomatic latent infection. This can range from days to years.[15] Various warning signs indicating acute and severe form of melioidosis is mentioned in Table 13.1.

Patients who usually develop septicaemic melioidosis usually have a short history of fever without clinically relevant focal infection. Most of the patients become severely ill within days; The blood cultures are likely to be positive in this condition. There may be associated metabolic acidosis that can lead to Kussmaul breathing. The patients may present with hypotension and signs of vital organ dysfunction. The radiologic

TABLE 13.1 Warning sign of melioidosis

- Acute high-grade fever
- Systemic symptoms (nausea, poor appetite, lethargy)
- Symptoms of pneumonia such as fever, respiratory distress, and cough
- Difficulty in breathing
- Shock (hypotension)

feature of consolidation of the lung may be present. There can be multi-focal patchy bilateral shadows that may or may not be associated with evolving abscess formation.

Some patients may have previous skin lesions that vary between superficial ery-thematous pustules and clusters of more profound violaceous skin eruptions. There may be a subcutaneous abscess in some patients. The visceral abscess in the liver, spleen, kid-ney, and prostate are common. Even meningitis can be present in the septicaemic patient.

Burkholderia disseminates hematogenously to various organs including subcuta-neous tissue, lymph nodes, the lungs, spleen, prostate, liver, kidney, skin, bone, and brain. Initially, multiple microscopic abscesses are formed, which spread bacteria in the circulation. The extent of such abscesses depends on the duration of the disease and comorbidity such as diabetes.

In the Darwin 30-year Prospective Melioidosis Study, a larger series of 1148 pri-mary melioidosis presentations, 1013 (88%) were acute, 106 (9%) were chronic, and 29 (3%) were considered to be activation of latent infection.[14] Septicaemic patients pro-gressed rapidly and presented with high fever with little or no cough.

On chest radiography, patients presenting with acute pneumonia might also have had lobar or multi-lobar involvement, necrotizing cavitations, or pleural effusion. In a study by Currie et al., 28% of *Burkholderia* pneumonia patients had multi-lobar involvement of the lungs. CT scans of the abdomen usually showed the abscess or involvement of the prostate, spleen, kidneys, and liver. In the Darwin study, pneumonia was the most common presentation of melioidosis (278 [51%] of 540 patients). Almost half of the cases had bacteraemia (55%). One hundred and sixteen (21%) patients devel-oped septic shock, out of which half of the patients died.[16] Blood cultures were positive for *B. pseudomallei* in 56% of a total of 1135 patients with a blood culture-confirmed septic shock occurred in 240 (21%) patients, usually on presentation or within 24 hours; 278 (24%) patients were managed in the ICU, 180 (16%) patients required mechanical ventilation, and 100 (9%) patients required renal replacement therapy.

In the multi-variate analysis, pneumonia was independently associated with various comorbidities like diabetes, cardiac failure, and chronic lung disease and presentation during the four high-rainfall months. Other risk factors of bacteraemia were the age of 50 years or above, heavy alcohol use, chronic kidney disease, immunosuppression, malig-nancy etc.[14] Nearly 75–87% of patients presenting with pneumonia or bacteraemia were expected to require ICU care.[17] Dermatological presentation is more common in children (60% of children versus 13% of adult cases), whereas pneumonia and bacteraemia are common in adults (54–59% versus 16–20% in children).[18] Brainstem encephalitis is a classical presentation of neurological melioidosis. The cranial nerves (mainly facial nerve) involvement and peripheral motor weakness were also common in neuromelioidosis.[16]

DIAGNOSIS

Melioidosis should be suspected in the appropriate clinic-epidemiological context (Table 13.2). The initial screening can be done by Gram stain of the appropriate clini-cal specimen. The organism is a gram-negative rod showing bipolar staining. Positive

TABLE 13.2 When to suspect?

- Known risk factors
- In the months of monsoon and epidemiological exposure to water or soil
  Without an immediately apparent aetiology, not responding to conventional
  antimicrobials like standard dosing regimens of β lactams, macrolides, or
  fluoroquinolones

Clinical presentation

- Pneumonia/septicaemia/deep-seated abscess (spleen, kidney, prostate, liver)
- Submandibular/cervical lymph node etc.
- Cutaneous lesion
  History of ulcerative/pustular cutaneous lesions in the recent past, unresponsive to
  conventional antimicrobials

Clinical correlations

- Previous culture reports, such as *Pseudomonas*, but having resistance to
  aminoglycosides, polymyxin, colistin, etc., which are practically discordant

blood or tissue cultures is the mainstay of diagnosis. Hence, obtaining blood cultures
and other tissue cultures (such as lymph node aspirate, pus from an abscess or cerebrospinal fluid, etc.) of all sick and suspected patients is essential. Species identification
of *B. pseudomallei* from culture growth can be ascertained by various methods like
i) conventional biochemical tests with triple-disc screening, ii) automated bacterial
identification systems, iii) immunoassays, iv) molecular identification by polymerase
chain reaction using *B. pseudomallei*-specific primers, and v) mass spectrometry.

A lateral flow immune (LFA) assay detecting *B. pseudomallei* specific capsular
polysaccharide (CPS), marketed under the name of Active Melioidosis Detect (AMD)
has the potential to reduce the time to diagnosis of melioidosis and is being used as a
point of care test.

DIFFERENTIAL DIAGNOSIS

Differential Diagnosis in ICU:

- a. Disseminated septic emboli
- b. Other Gram-negative sepsis/bacteraemia
- c. Staphylococcal bacteraemia
- d. Invasive pneumococcal disease
- e. Necrotizing fasciitis
- f. Invasive meningococcal disease
- g. Leptospirosis
- h. Plague

    i. Malaria
    j. Enteric fever
    k. Typhus
    l. Vibrio vulnificus infection

GUIDING FACTORS FOR EMPIRIC ANTIBIOTIC IN ENDEMIC MELIOIDOSIS

The choice of empirical antibiotic therapy should be based on the probable causative organism in a particular geographical location in a septic patient before the blood culture result is available. Uncontrolled diabetes, renal failure, and immunological status also guide the choice of antibiotics.

TREATMENT

Treating septicaemic melioidosis is challenging due to difficulties in identifying the bacteria. Clinical suspicion of the organism should be made based on the risk factors and clinical presentation. Along with antibiotics, controlling the source, such as drainage of the abscess, should be done if feasible. It is crucial as a part of treating as well as preventing treatment failures, especially in septic joints and prostatic collection.

Antibiotics

Intensive Therapy: Antibiotics can be initiated as soon as possible per sepsis management guidelines. One should prefer to start meropenem or ceftazidime depending on the choices and as per the 2020 revised *Darwin Melioidosis Treatment Guidelines.*[19] Four weeks is required for pneumonia with lymphadenopathy or ICU admission or deep-seated collection (abscess anywhere other than skin), 6 weeks for osteomyelitis, and 8 weeks for central nervous system or arterial infection.[20] The details of antibiotics are discussed in Chapter 9 on drug management

Fluid Management

As per the *Surviving Sepsis Campaign* 2021 guidelines, patients presenting with sepsis-induced hypoperfusion and septic shock, initial fluid resuscitation should be done with 30 ml/kg crystalloids. Subsequent fluid therapy should be guided by dynamic intravascular volume and organ perfusion parameters such as cardiac output monitoring, stroke volume variation, pulse pressure variation, passive leg raise test, etc.

Vasopressor

Vasopressors should be added in cases of persistent hypotension during or after adequate initial fluid resuscitation. The target mean arterial pressure is 65 mm Hg. Norepinephrine is the initial vasopressor of choice.

Ventilation

Patients having acute hypoxemic failure may be managed with high-flow nasal oxygen. If invasive mechanical ventilation is indicated, patients should be managed with lung protective ventilation with a low tidal volume of 4–8 ml per kg of predicted body weight and a plateau pressure goal of 30 cm H_2O or less. Other supportive ICU care for melioidosis remains the same as for critically ill septic patients.

PROGNOSIS

Relapses are common in melioidosis patients with inadequate treatment and in patients with severe melioidosis, multi-focal abscesses, prolonged bacteraemia, and poor compliance. The mortality has been up to 50% in acute fulminant melioidosis patients.[16] With early diagnosis and administration of timely appropriate antibiotics (meropenem or ceftazidime), and access to high-quality ICU care, the general mortality of melioidosis could be reduced from 90% to less than 10%.[14]

CONCLUSIONS

The use of initial empiric antibiotics should be based on the high likelihood of a particular organism and the severity of illness, including associated shock. The site of infection involvement, likely organisms for these sites, history of past antibiotic use/failure, associated co-morbid condition, and local microbiology data should be considered in deciding on empiric antimicrobial therapy. Antibiotics can be modified as per Gram stain and blood/tissue aspirate culture report whenever the report is available.

REFERENCES

1. Reinhart K, et al. Recognizing Sepsis as a Global Health Priority – A WHO Resolution. N Engl J Med 2017; 377(5): 414–7.
2. Fay K, et al. Assessment of Health Care Exposures and Outcomes in Adult Patients with Sepsis and Septic Shock. JAMA Netw Open 2020; 3(7): e206004.

3. Martínez ML, et al. Impact of Source Control in Patients with Severe Sepsis and Septic Shock. Crit Care Med 2017; 45(1): 11–19.
4. Chaowagul W, et al. Melioidosis: A Major Cause of Community-Acquired Septicemia in Northeastern Thailand. J Infect Dis 1989; 159(5): 890–99.
5. Douglas MW, et al. Epidemiology of Community-Acquired and Nosocomial Bloodstream Infections in Tropical Australia: A 12-Month Prospective Study. Trop Med Int Health 2004; 9(7): 795–804.
6. Novosad SA, et al. Vital Signs: Epidemiology of Sepsis: Prevalence of Health Care Factors and Opportunities for Prevention. MMWR Morb Mortal Wkly Rep 2016; 65(33): 864–9.
7. Vincent JL, et al. International Study of the Prevalence and Outcomes of Infection in Intensive Care Units. JAMA 2009; 302(21): 2323–9.
8. Toh V, et al. Clinical Characteristics and Predictors of Mortality in Patients with Melioidosis: The Kapit Experience. Trop Med Int Health 2021; 26(6): 664–71.
9. Evans L, et al. Surviving Sepsis Campaign: International Guidelines for Management of Sepsis and Septic Shock 2021. Intensive Care Med 2021; 47(11): 1181–247.
10. Singer M, et al. The Third International Consensus Definitions for Sepsis and Septic Shock (Sepsis-3). JAMA 2016; 315(8): 801–10.
11. Minne L, et al. Evaluation of SOFA-Based Models for Predicting Mortality in the ICU: A Systematic Review. Crit Care 2008; 12(6): R161.
12. Levy MM, et al. The Surviving Sepsis Campaign Bundle: 2018 Update. Intensive Care Med 2018; 44(6): 925–28.
13. De Backer D, et al. Septic Shock: A Microcirculation Disease. Curr Opin Anaesthesiol 2021; 34(2): 85–91.
14. Currie BJ, et al. The Darwin Prospective Melioidosis Study: A 30-Year Prospective, Observational Investigation. Lancet Infect Dis 2021 (12): 1737–1746.
15. Currie BJ, et al. Melioidosis: Acute and Chronic Disease, Relapse and Re-Activation. Trans R Soc Trop Med Hyg 2000; 94(3): 301–4.
16. Currie BJ, et al. The Epidemiology and Clinical Spectrum of Melioidosis: 540 Cases from the 20 Year Darwin Prospective Study. PLoS Negl Trop Dis 2010; 4(11): e900.
17. Stephens DP, et al. Melioidosis Causing Critical Illness: A Review of 24 Years of Experience from the Royal Darwin Hospital ICU. Crit Care Med 2016; 44(8): 1500–5.
18. McLeod C, et al. Clinical Presentation and Medical Management of Melioidosis in Children: A 24-Year Prospective Study in the Northern Territory of Australia and Review of the Literature. Clin Infect Dis 2015; 60(1): 21–6.
19. Sullivan RP, et al. 2020 Review and Revision of the 2015 Darwin Melioidosis Treatment Guideline; Paradigm Drift Not Shift. PLoS Negl Trop Dis 2020; 14(9): e0008659.
20. Pitman MC, et al. Intravenous Therapy Duration and Outcomes in Melioidosis: A New Treatment Paradigm. PLoS Negl Trop Dis 2015; 9(3): e0003586.

Cutaneous Melioidosis

14

Chandra Sekhar Sirka

Department of Dermatology & Venereology, All India Institute of Medical Sciences, Bhubaneswar, India

Arpita Nibedita Rout

Department of Dermatology & Venereology, All India Institute of Medical Sciences, Bhubaneswar, India

Prasanta R Mohapatra

Department of Pulmonary Medicine and Critical Care, All India Institute of Medical Sciences, Bhubaneswar, India

Contents

EPIDEMIOLOGY

Cutaneous melioidosis (CM) is usually localized and belongs to less severe forms among the type of melioidosis. CM is found in almost 10–25% of affected adults and as high as 60% of paediatric patients.[1,2] Primary forms of CM are more common.[1] CM is probably the second most common presentation in children.

DOI: 10.1201/9781003324010-14

TABLE 14.1 Comparison of skin manifestation by regions[1,2]

COUNTRY/REGIONS	NO./TOTAL (%)
Australia	123/761 (16)
Malaysia	99/402 (25)
Singapore	65/372 (17)
India	23/180 (13)
Thailand	35/247 (14)

MODE OF TRANSMISSION

The bacteria *Burkholderia pseudomallei* are usually present in soil and water in the endemic areas (Table 14.1). The history of travel to endemic countries is therefore important, especially in cases reported from non-endemic areas.

The skin infection is usually acquired through skin inoculation or contamination of wounds. Skin inoculation is possible while working in rice fields with abrasions or open wounds, walking barefoot, and bathing in natural rainwater ponds.[3] In endemic areas, a small traumatic injury to the skin with a small open wound may become contaminated during the rainy season, while walking in mud, or from water and soil in the endemic areas, leading to skin and soft-tissue infection initially, and may progress to involve the underlying deep tissue. However, when there are multiple pustular lesions, it is possible to involve different sites due to hematogenous spread. This hematogenous spread is uncommon in cutaneous melioidosis.[4,5]

The incubation period is around 3 weeks.[2] Immunocompromised hosts are at higher risk of developing an infection after exposure, such as those with diabetes mellitus, heavy alcohol consumption, chronic kidney, liver, and lung disease, and thalassemia.[6–8] The most common of these is diabetes. Primary CM is possible without any risk factors, as discussed in other chapters.

CLINICAL PRESENTATION

Two forms of CM have been distinguished: primary, the infection first starting on the skin, and secondary, in which cutaneous infection results from spread from some extracutaneous location.[2] In chronic CM, the lesion duration exceeds 2 months.[2]

The primary form is more common, accounting for about 88% of cases in one literature review.[2] Primary CM is often localized, and bacteraemia is rare.[7] People having direct exposure to *B. pseudomallei* are more likely to have primary CM. It usually presents as a skin nodule after blunt trauma. The lesion may have tenderness but with no sign of inflammation. The cutaneous form may be rarely associated with lymphadenopathy or fever. There may not be any fever or other systemic symptoms in some cases.

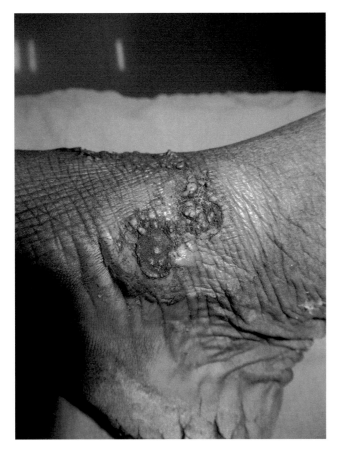

FIGURE 14.1 Multiple superficial ulcers covered with brownish black crusts over the malleolar area with multiple papules in the surrounding skin.

Therefore, it may be easily misdiagnosed as a non-infectious lesion. Almost one-third of such cases can have chronic infection.[2]

The most common cutaneous presentation is an abscess, seen in around 58% of cases.[2] Other forms that have been described are cellulitis, ulcers, and nodules[9] (Figure 14.1). Multiple-site involvement and multiple cutaneous forms in the same patient have also been reported. Cutaneous lesions are rarely an extension of underlying infection, such as chronic melioidosis, osteomyelitis, or lymphadenitis. The common sites affected are lower limbs, head and neck, upper limbs, and trunk.[2]

The primary form may be associated with necrotizing fasciitis and soft-tissue abscess, including deep-organ abscesses, as reported in Southeast Asia.[10–12] There has been a report of melioidosis associated with polyarteritis nodosa.[6] Other manifestations are single pustules, boils, dry asymmetric erythematous flat lesions, and crusted erythematous lesions. Disseminated and septic melioidosis may be associated with extensive skin pustules and ecthyma-like lesions in secondary forms.[11] Secondary CM can also present with Sweet syndrome-like lesions.[13]

The children of Cambodia and Thailand frequently had skin and soft tissue involvement, along with suppurative parotitis or cervical lymphadenopathy.[14] Erythema nodosum, classically seen as tender erythematous subcutaneous nodules, may be an unusual form. It could be a delayed hypersensitivity reaction triggered by melioidosis infection.[15]

Lungs are the most common extracutaneous site to be affected and are involved in up to one in four patients.[2] Recrudescence of skin melioidosis is uncommon.

Melioidosis can also present to dermatologists in the setting of prolonged use of systemic steroids and other immunosuppressives, often used for various chronic cutaneous conditions. Such patients are at higher risk of developing features of dissemination or septicemia.[16]

DIFFERENTIAL DIAGNOSIS

With a wide spectrum of cutaneous presentations, differential diagnoses like fungal infections, tuberculosis, and atypical mycobacterial infections are possible. Other diseases like lymphogranuloma venereum, tularaemia, and cat scratch disease have similar clinical and histological presentations. Even superadded streptococcal and staphylococcal infections are possible and should also be considered.

DIAGNOSIS

Confirming the diagnosis is challenging. More than 90% of patients have localized disease, and only about 2% are reported to be bacteremic.[17] The demonstration of the bacterium by Gram staining and culture of the skin lesions or from histology should be done as practicable. The skin manifestation of disseminated melioidosis may be a clue to early diagnosis by Gram staining pus from skin pustules. Occasionally, the organism can also be seen within macrophages and giant cells in the prolonged forms of cutaneous melioidosis.

TREATMENT

The infection is associated with subcutaneous-or-deeper tissue involvement and should be treated successfully by incision and drainage of the abscess, along with appropriate antibiotic therapy using ceftazidime or meropenem discussed in Chapter 9 on drug management.

Primary skin melioidosis is usually localized and rarely fatal. Melioidosis is a disease with a broad spectrum of dermatological and other clinical presentations. Clinicians in endemic regions should have a low threshold to consider melioidosis. In endemic countries, melioidosis must be considered a differential diagnosis of nodular or ulcerative cutaneous lesions.

REFERENCES

1. Gassiep I, et al. Human Melioidosis. Clin Microbiol Rev 2020; 33(2): e00006–19.
2. Fertitta L, et al. Cutaneous Melioidosis: A Review of the Literature. Int J Dermatol 2019; 58(2): 221–27.
3. Limmathurotsakul D, et al. Activities of Daily Living Associated with Acquisition of Melioidosis in Northeast Thailand: A Matched Case-Control Study. PLoS Negl Trop Dis 2013; 7(2): e2072.
4. Sridharan S, et al. Melioidosis in Critical Care: A Review. Indian J Crit Care Med 2021; 25(Suppl 2): S161–65.
5. Gibney KB, et al. Cutaneous Melioidosis in the Tropical Top End of Australia: A Prospective Study and Review of the Literature. Clin Infect Dis 2008; 47(5): 603–9.
6. Suputtamongkol Y, et al. Risk Factors for Melioidosis and Bacteremic Melioidosis. Clin Infect Dis 1999; 29(2): 408–13.
7. Currie BJ, et al. Endemic Melioidosis in Tropical Northern Australia: A 10-Year Prospective Study and Review of the Literature. Clin Infect Dis 2000; 31(4): 981–6.
8. Meumann EM, et al. Clinical Features and Epidemiology of Melioidosis Pneumonia: Results from a 21-Year Study and Review of the Literature. Clin Infect Dis 2012; 54(3): 362–9.
9. Tran D, et al. Cutaneous Melioidosis. Clin Exp Dermatol 2002; 27(4): 280–2.
10. Teo L, et al. Cutaneous Melioidosis. J Eur Acad Dermatol Venereol 2006; 20(10): 1322–4.
11. Apisarnthanarak A, et al. Photo Quiz. A Thai Woman with Fever and Skin Lesions. Clin Infect Dis 2005; 40(7): 988–9, 1053–4.
12. Wang YS, et al. Cutaneous Melioidosis and Necrotizing Fasciitis Caused by *Burkholderia pseudomallei*. Emerg Infect Dis 2003; 9(11): 1484–5.
13. Vithoosan S, et al. A Rare Case of Sweet Syndrome Secondary to Melioidosis. BMC Dermatol 2019; 19(1): 16.
14. Turner P, et al. A Retrospective Analysis of Melioidosis in Cambodian Children, 2009–2013. BMC Infect Dis 2016; 16(1): 688.
15. Tan PY, et al. Erythema Nodosum – An Atypical Presentation of Melioidosis. Rev Soc Bras Med Trop 2022; 55: e00362022.
16. Pradhan S, et al. Melioidosis Complicating Lepromatous Leprosy with Type 2 Lepra Reaction: A Rare Case Report from India. Lepr Rev 2019; 90: 450–5.
17. Currie BJ, et al. The Darwin Prospective Melioidosis Study: A 30-Year Prospective, Observational Investigation. Lancet Infect Dis 2021 (12): 1737–1746.

Cardiac Melioidosis

15

Rama Chandra Barik
Department of Cardiology, All India Institute of Medical Sciences, Bhubaneswar, India

Rudra Pratap Mahapatra
Department of Cardiothoracic and Vascular Surgery, All India Institute of Medical Sciences, Bhubaneswar, India

Contents

INTRODUCTION

The cardiovascular manifestations of melioidosis are rare compared to other more common complications like pneumonia and intra-abdominal infections.[1–3] In the absence of more extensive case studies, the true epidemiology of cardiac melioidosis is unknown.

It is fascinating to recollect Whitmore's description of small vegetation on the mitral valve, which was due to infective endocarditis caused by *Burkholderia pseudomallei*, in the post-mortem examination of an intravenous morphia abuser.[4]

DOI: 10.1201/9781003324010-15

TABLE 15.1   Cardiovascular manifestations due to *Burkholderia pseudomallei*[4-14]

CARDIAC COMPLICATIONS	REMARKS
• Pericarditis • Endocarditis • Myocarditis • Prosthetic valve infection • Pacemaker pocket infection	Usual complications
Congestive heart failure (CHF)	CHF increases the risk of cardiac melioidosis
Vascular • Embolism • Aneurysm • Thrombosis • Portal vein thrombosis	Arteries of Intracranial vessels, coronary arteries, abdominal aorta, subclavian artery, and iliac artery

Chapter 2 on epidemiology in this book describes the risk factors of melioidosis. The cardiovascular manifestations (table 15.1) and summary of cases (table 15.2) of melioidosis are discussed.

PERICARDITIS

Pericarditis is the most common cardiac complication, followed by myocardial abscess and endocarditis.[5,6] Pericardial effusion occurs in 1–3% of patients with melioidosis, mainly reported in the endemic regions.[7] In the *Darwin Prospective Melioidosis Study* from Australia, only 4 out of 540 (<1%) documented cases had pericarditis.[8] In most cases of pericarditis, the presentations have been sub-acute to chronic, mimicking tubercular pericardial effusion.[9]

ENDOCARDITIS

It is rare (~1%) and is rarely reported in the literature.[10,11]

MYOCARDITIS

Three cases have been reported. Two of three patients died of embolism or extracardiac abscess.[5]

TABLE 15.2 List of some reported cases of cardiovascular melioidosis

AUTHOR, YEAR, COUNTRY	AGE (YEARS), SEX	COMPLICATION	SYSTEMS AFFECTED	TREATMENT	OUTCOME
Lu et al. (2018), Malaysia	38, Male	Constrictive pericarditis	Cardiovascular	IV ceftazidime, IV meropenem, oral bactrim, IV ciprofloxacin	Complication
Direksunthorn (2017), Thailand	54, Male	Portal vein thrombosis	Cardiovascular	IV ceftazidime, IV metronidazole, oral amoxicillin-clavulanic acid	Recovery
Li et al. (2015), Hong Kong	82, Male	Mycotic aneurysm of the aortic arch/left subclavian artery	Cardiovascular	IV amoxicillin-clavulanate and azithromycin, IV ceftazidime, oral amoxicillin-clavulanate and doxycycline, IV meropenem and doxycycline, IV minocycline and moxifloxacin	Mortality
Abidin et al. (2007), 65, Male		Pacemaker infection	Others	IV ampicillin-sulbactam, IV meropenem, IV ceftazidime, oral TMP-SMX, and doxycycline	Recovery
Mohammad and Ghazali (2017), Malaysia	64, Male	Venous thrombo-embolism and cavitary pneumonia	Cardiovascular and Respiratory	IV ceftazidime and IV heparin	Recovery
Schindler et al. (2002), United States	58, Male	Infected intrathoracic subclavian artery and pseudoaneurysm	Cardiovascular	Coronary artery bypass grafting procedure and pseudoaneurysm repair, femoro-femoral bypass graft, IV ceftazidime, oral doxycycline and amoxicillin clavulanic acid	Recovery
Chung et al (2008), Taiwan	73, Male	Cardiac tamponade	Cardiovascular	**Induction therapy**: A 14-day course of ceftazidime alone **Eradication therapy:** TMP-SMX, doxycycline and chloramphenicol	Recovery
Majid et al. (1990), Australia	35, Male	Pericardial melioidosis	Cardiovascular	Antibiotics, successful surgical management	Recovery

(Continued)

TABLE 15.2 List of some reported cases of cardiovascular melioidosis (*Continued*)

AUTHOR, YEAR, COUNTRY	AGE (YEARS), SEX	COMPLICATION	SYSTEMS AFFECTED	TREATMENT	OUTCOME
Lu et al. (2018), Malaysia	38, Male	Constrictive pericarditis	Cardiovascular	IV ceftazidime 2 gm, 6-hourly IV meropenem 1 gm, 8-hourly, in combination with oral bactrim (trimethoprim/sulphamethoxazole 80/400 mg) twice daily	
Schultze et al. (2012), Switzerland	44, Male	Pericardial effusion	Cardiovascular	Ceftazidime 2 g every 6 hours for 2 weeks followed by three-month maintenance treatment with doxycycline, trimethoprim-sulfamethoxazole, and leucovorine	Recovery
Elsharabassy et al. (2021), Germany	19, Male	Pericardial effusion	Cardiovascular	IV meropenem for 2 weeks and was discharged with cotrimoxazole orally as maintenance therapy	Recovered
Sivaradjy et al (2021), India	65, Male	Pericardial effusion	Cardiovascular	Injection ceftazidime twice daily	Recovered

VASCULITIS

It manifests as a mycotic or pseudoaneurysm of the large and medium-sized arteries.[12,13]

PACEMAKER POCKET INFECTION[14]

Infection of a pacemaker secondary to *B. pseudomallei* is relatively rare but can be a severe complication of any implanted intracardiac device. Early diagnosis and appropriate treatment with culture-sensitive antibiotics are crucial for treating cardiac melioidosis.[14]

CONGESTIVE HEART FAILURE

Congestive heart failure has been considered a risk factor for cardiovascular melioidosis.[8]

More than 9% of reported cases of cardiac melioidosis are males. Its overall mortality of 18% varies significantly depending on cardiac involvement. The mortality has been high in myocarditis and low in pericarditis. With *B. pseudomallei,* only about 10% of patients with pericarditis succumbed, compared to 17% of patients with endocarditis and 100% with myocarditis. This high mortality is based on post-mortem, although most patients with myocarditis were diagnosed post-mortem. Most of the patients with endocarditis are under-reported due to the smaller size of valvular vegetation. Most of the reported sub-centimetre vegetations did not require valvular replacement. In addition to intensive intravenous antibiotics, a prolonged course of oral eradication antibiotic therapy is needed for undiagnosed endocarditis.[3]

REFERENCES

1. Currie BJ, et al. The Darwin Prospective Melioidosis Study: A 30-Year Prospective, Observational Investigation. Lancet Infect Dis 2021; 21(12): 1737–46.
2. Meumann EM, et al. Clinical Features and Epidemiology of Melioidosis Pneumonia: Results from a 21-Year Study and Review of the Literature. Clin Infect Dis 2012; 54(3): 362–9.
3. Velusamy R, et al. Melioidosis and the Heart: A Systematic Review. Trop Med Infect Dis 2020; 5(3):121. https://doi.org/10.3390/tropicalmed5030121
4. Whitmore A. An Account of a Glanders-Like Disease Occurring in Rangoon. J Hyg (Lond) 1913; 13(1): 1–34.

5. Baumann BB, et al. Systemic Melioidosis Presenting as Myocardial Infarct. Ann Intern Med 1967; 67(4): 836–42.
6. Birnie E, et al. Global Burden of Melioidosis in 2015: A Systematic Review and Data Synthesis. Lancet Infect Dis 2019; 19(8): 892–902.
7. Kuruvilla TS, et al. Melioidotic Pericardial Effusion. Indian J Med Sci 2010; 64(2): 94–8.
8. Currie BJ, et al. The Epidemiology and Clinical Spectrum of Melioidosis: 540 Cases from the 20 Year Darwin Prospective Study. PLoS Negl Trop Dis 2010; 4(11): e900.
9. Chetchotisakd P, et al. Melioidosis Pericarditis Mimicking Tuberculous Pericarditis. Clin Infect Dis 2010; 51(5): e46–9.
10. Subramony H, et al. Disseminated Melioidosis with Native Valve Endocarditis: A Case Report. Eur Heart J Case Rep 2019; 3(2): ytz097. https://doi.org/10.1093/ehjcr/ytz097
11. Piyasiri LB, et al. Endocarditis in Melioidosis. Ceylon Med J 2016; 61(4): 192–3.
12. Restrepo CS, et al. Infected ("Mycotic") Coronary Artery Aneurysm: Systematic Review. J Cardiovasc Comput Tomogr 2020; 14(6): e99–104.
13. Rao J, et al. Abdominal Aortic Pseudoaneurysm Secondary to Melioidosis. Asian J Surg 2009; 32(1): 64–9.
14. Zainal Abidin I, et al. Pacemaker Infection Secondary to *Burkholderia pseudomallei*. Pacing Clin Electrophysiol 2007; 30(11): 1420–2.

Melioidosis of Bone and Joint

16

Sujit Kumar Tripathy

Department of Orthopaedics, All India Institute of Medical Sciences, Bhubaneswar, India

Mantu Jain

Department of Orthopaedics, All India Institute of Medical Sciences, Bhubaneswar, India

Narayan Prasad Mishra

Department of Orthopaedics, All India Institute of Medical Sciences, Bhubaneswar, India

Contents

INTRODUCTION

Melioidosis is caused by the Gram-negative bacteria *Burkholderia pseudomallei*. This pathogen's infection of the bone and joints is uncommon, but it can lead to severe consequences unless diagnosed and intervened appropriately.[1–4] The knee joints are more

DOI: 10.1201/9781003324010-16

commonly involved, followed by the ankle, hip, and shoulder joints.[5] The diagnosis is often missed or delayed because of a lack of awareness, diagnostic facility, and non-specific clinical features. The clinical, radiological, and histological features of bone and joint melioidosis mimic many other diseases, and the major challenge is to differentiate it from tuberculosis.[3–5] Melioidosis should be the first differential diagnosis for bone and joint infection in patients returning from the endemic zone.

EPIDEMIOLOGY

Melioidotic bone and joint infections are endemic in Southeast Asia and Northern Australia. A study from Northern Australia found that bone and joint infection incidence in melioidosis is 7.6%,[2,4] while another study from Thailand reported it to be 14–27%.[1,6] The incidence of osteoarticular infection in these patients was 29%, as reported by a study from Brunei.[7] A study from Christian Medical College Vellore, India, reported a 9.2% incidence of musculoskeletal involvement among melioidosis patients.[8]

PATHOGENESIS

Bone and joint infection of *B. pseudomallei* occurs via direct inoculation through minor skin abrasions, wound infections, and abscesses or through hematogenous spread in patients with a primary diagnosis of melioidotic pneumonia or septicaemia.[5] This infection is usually linked to occupational and recreational exposure to surface water, landscaping, and gardening in endemic areas. This is more common in males as they are more exposed to *B. pseudomallei* while working in rice paddies and as they are involved in other outdoor activities. Diabetes mellitus, hypertension, chronic kidney disease, malignancies, prolonged corticosteroid use, and heavy alcohol consumption are the various risk factors for the disease.[2,4,5] Studies reported a 100-fold increased risk of melioidosis among diabetic patients.[1–4] The underlying comorbidities lead to immune dysfunction like impaired polymorphonuclear phagocyte function; thus, phagocytic cells fail to clear the pathogenic organism from the body. One study found a 5.7 times increased risk of septic arthritis among melioidotic patients with associated diabetes mellitus, systemic lupus erythematosus, and chronic renal failure.[6] In their series of 50 musculoskeletal melioidotic patients, Shetty et al. reported that 80% of patients had one or more comorbidities, and diabetes was the most common.[9]

CLINICAL FEATURES

The melioidotic bone and joint infection usually manifests as septic arthritis, osteomyelitis, or soft-tissue abscess. However, the clinical presentations of these entities are not distinguishable from the infections by common organisms such as *Staphylococcus*, *Streptococcus*, and others; thus, it often leads to delays in diagnosis.[2,5] As a general rule, melioidosis should be considered in the differential diagnosis of bone and joint infections in patients from the endemic areas and among the travelers of non-endemic areas who have recently travelled to the endemic zone.

Melioidosis can involve single or multiple bones and joints. Septic arthritis and osteomyelitis patients usually present with localized pain, swelling, redness, warmth, and a decreased range of movement of the affected joint. The presentation is usually subacute or chronic, and the fever is usually persistent without associated shock or respiratory failure. Perumal et al. from India reported that 60% of their patients presented with symptoms of >6 weeks.[8] The overall mortality is low in these bone and joint infections compared to other forms of the disease.[3,4]

A study from Australia revealed that melioidotic septic arthritis and osteomyelitis were the primary presentations in 25.4% of patients (16/63 episodes) and 31.7% of patients (20/63 episodes) of melioidosis (20/63 episodes).[9] Multi-focal infection was observed in >50% of their patients (32/50).[9] Teparrakkul et al. from Thailand reported 14.43% of musculoskeletal melioidosis in their series of 679 patients.[1] The knees are the most commonly affected joints, followed by the ankle, hip, and shoulder. Contrary to this, Kosuwon et al. reported the shoulder as the more commonly affected joint.[6] In melioidotic osteomyelitis, the femur and tibia are more commonly affected than the upper-limb bones. Apart from these, few cases of infective spondylodiscitis have been reported due to melioidosis, and it mimics tubercular spondylodiscitis.[6]

DIAGNOSIS

Lack of awareness, limited resources to isolate the organism, and similarity in the clinical presentation of the disease with other infectious diseases such as tuberculosis have made diagnosing melioidosis very challenging. The gold standard in the diagnosis of osteoarticular melioidosis is the isolation of *B. psudomallei* from the specimens collected from infected bones, intervertebral discs, or fluid aspirated from the septic joints. Wu et al. from China reported that blood was the most frequent clinical sample where *B. pseudomallei* was isolated in their series, accounting for 93.2% of cases. It was consistent with the recommendation of previous literature that blood samples should be collected whenever there is any suspicion of melioidotic osteomyelitis and septic arthritis.[10] A positive blood culture with positive radiological findings (particularly computerized tomography [CT] images) nearly ascertains the diagnosis of bone and joint melioidosis. However, needle aspiration of the abscess, necrotic lesion of the bone or the bone marrow, tissue materials from ulcers and wounds, and tissue from the discitis lesion site should also be collected, transported, and handled appropriately by skilled personnel to isolate the organism with minimal failure.[2,5]

Radiological tools such as plain X-ray and CT scans help to suspect melioidotic osteomyelitis preoperative diagnosis. Plain radiographs show cortical irregularity and thickening with subchondral sclerosis (Figure 16.1A). Magnetic resonance imaging

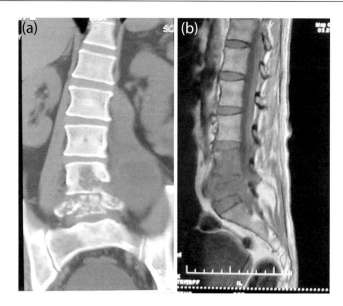

FIGURE 16.1   A 62-year-old man presented with back pain, low-grade fever, and neurological deficit. The radiograph showed superior end-plate erosion of the L5 vertebra with L4/L5 vertebral body involvement (a). Magnetic resonance imaging confirmed soft-tissue collection around the L4/L5 vertebra with articular erosion and L4 and L5 vertebral bodies involvement (b).

(MRI) of the affected bone and joints can be used to detect both osteomyelitis and septic arthritis. MRI reveals joint effusion, erosion of the articular surfaces, bone marrow, and surrounding muscle oedema (Figure 16.1B). A three-phase 99m technetium scan shows increased uptake in the affected joints. Histopathological examination of the intraoperative samples may show acute supportive inflammation consistent with pyogenic infection or a granulomatous lesion resembling a tubercular lesion. Molecular methods like polymerase chain reaction have less sensitivity than blood, fluid, or tissue specimen culture results. Still, they can be used as a diagnostic tool.[11]

TREATMENT

Treatment of melioidotic bone and joint infections includes containment of infection with surgery and appropriate antibiotics. Patients with unifocal disease of the long bone without abscess formation and vertebral osteomyelitis usually respond to non-surgical treatment.[9] However, aggressive surgical treatment is warranted when there is an abscess or septic arthritis formation, extensive bone necrosis, or if there is no response to initial antibiotic therapy. The treatment in such a condition includes extensive debridement of infected bones, arthrotomy, and lavage of involved joints, along with administration of systemic antibiotics active against *B. pseudomallei*. There should be repeated wound debridement and need infected tissue removal to ward off the infection.[8,9] The principles of treatment in melioidotic osteomyelitis are the same as that for other conditions, such as adequate drainage, extensive debridement of all necrotic tissue, dead-space management, and soft-tissue coverage, and restoration of the blood supply. The patient's general condition must be considered before deciding on the surgical treatment's aggressiveness. Many surgeons resort to the antibiotic application (PMMA beads) to eradicate the infection in long-standing cases.[8,9]

The antibiotic treatment should be continued along with or after surgical debridement with appropriate serial inflammatory-marker monitoring. The antibiotic treatment protocol is initial intensive therapy with high dose intravenous ceftazidime, meropenem, or imipenem, followed by maintenance therapy with high dose oral trimethoprim-sulfamethoxazole (TMP-SMZ).[5] For deep-seated infections and complications, intravenous antibiotics should be continued for a minimum of 4 weeks, followed by oral antibiotics for a minimum of 6 months.[12] Inflammatory markers and clinical signs of improvement are used to monitor the response of the disease to a specific therapy. Ceftazidime is the drug of choice in intensive treatment. Oral antibiotics like amoxicillin-clavulanic acid, cotrimoxazole, meropenem, and doxycycline may occasionally be used as alternative maintenance therapy. It is crucial to complete the treatment, including eradication therapy, to prevent relapse in melioidosis. Shetty et al. reported relapse in 10 patients with melioidotic bone and joint infections. Seven of these 10 patients had received <4 weeks of antibiotics.[9] The average time between discharge and relapse was nearly 21 weeks. A higher relapse rate of 30% has been reported if the overall duration of antimicrobial therapy is less than 8 weeks.[13] The relapse should be considered and treated as a first episode. Unfortunately, no specific vaccine is available for melioidosis.

CONCLUSION

There is a rising trend of *B. pseudomallei*-induced bone and joint infections both in the endemic and non-endemic zones. An early diagnosis and treatment can reduce morbidity and mortality. Isolation of the organism from the lesional fluid, tissue, or blood is considered the gold standard for diagnosis. The collection, transportation, and handling of the specimen must be performed judiciously. Treatment consists of antimicrobial therapy coupled with aggressive surgical debridement until all the necrotic tissues are removed. Appropriate antibiotic doses and duration must be completed to prevent disease relapse.

REFERENCES

1. Teparrakkul P, et al. Rheumatological Manifestations in Patients with Melioidosis. Southeast Asian J Trop Med Public Health 2008; 39(4): 649–55.
2. Currie BJ, et al. The Epidemiology and Clinical Spectrum of Melioidosis: 540 Cases from the 20 Year Darwin Prospective Study. PLoS Negl Trop Dis 2010; 4(11): e900.

3. Parameswaran U, et al. Melioidosis at Royal Darwin Hospital in the Big 2009–2010 Wet Season: Comparison with the Preceding 20 Years. Med J Aust 2012; 196(5): 345–8.

4. Currie BJ, et al. Endemic Melioidosis in Tropical Northern Australia: A 10-Year Prospective Study and Review of the Literature. Clin Infect Dis 2000; 31(4): 981–6.

5. Raja NS, et al. *Burkholderia pseudomallei* Causing Bone and Joint Infections: A Clinical Update. Infect Dis Ther 2016; 5(1): 17–29.

6. Kosuwon W, et al. Melioidotic Septic Arthritis and its Risk Factors. J Bone Joint Surg Am 2003; 85(6): 1058–61.

7. Pande KC, et al. Melioidosis of the Extremities in Brunei Darussalam. Singapore Med J 2011; 52(5): 346–50.

8. Perumal R, et al. Melioidosis of the Musculoskeletal System. Med Princ Pract 2020; 29(2): 121–27.

9. Shetty RP, et al. Management of Melioidosis Osteomyelitis and Septic Arthritis. Bone Joint J 2015; 97-b(2): 277–82.

10. Wu H, et al. Osteomyelitis and Septic Arthritis Due to *Burkholderia pseudomallei*: A 10-Year Retrospective Melioidosis Study from South China. Front Cell Infect Microbiol 2021; 11: 654745.

11. Richardson LJ, et al. Towards a Rapid Molecular Diagnostic for Melioidosis: Comparison of DNA Extraction Methods from Clinical Specimens. J Microbiol Methods 2012; 88(1): 179–81.

12. Sullivan RP, et al. 2020 Review and Revision of the 2015 Darwin Melioidosis Treatment Guideline; Paradigm Drift Not Shift. PLoS Negl Trop Dis 2020; 14(9): e0008659.

13. Chaowagul W, et al. Relapse in Melioidosis: Incidence and Risk Factors. J Infect Dis 1993; 168(5): 1181–5.

Prevention of Melioidosis

17

Prasanta R Mohapatra
Department of Pulmonary Medicine and Critical Care,
All India Institute of Medical Sciences, Bhubaneswar, India

Baijayantimala Mishra
Department of Microbiology, All India Institute
of Medical Sciences, Bhubaneswar, India

Contents

INTRODUCTION

Melioidosis is caused by a saprophytic Gram-negative bacillus called *Burkholderia pseudomallei*, which remains in the soil and water of hot and humid regions within

DOI: 10.1201/9781003324010-17

tropical countries. The disease classically presents as an acute manifestation of pneumonia, sepsis, and multi-organ abscesses. If untreated, it has a very high mortality rate.

GLOBAL BURDEN

The projected global burden of melioidosis is more than 4.6 million disability-adjusted life-years (DALYs) and is more than many other tropical diseases.[1] Melioidosis mostly affects poverty-stricken rural people; more than 99% of deaths due to melioidosis happen in low-income countries.[2] Hot and humid weather, unprotected barefoot workers in rice fields, and unprotected civil construction workers are predisposed to the added burden and spread of melioidosis.[3] The actual incidence of melioidosis is much more common in tropical countries in Southeast Asia and other regions than ever reported. Therefore, infection prevention is the key strategy to prevent melioidosis.

CURRENT GAPS IN KNOWLEDGE AND LABORATORY INFRASTRUCTURE AND PREVENTION

Lack of awareness among doctors on the clinical manifestation of the disease leads to misdiagnosis of the suspected cases. Secondly, the wide-ranging clinical presentation mimics other diseases, such as tuberculosis, ultimately delaying the diagnosis. Many samples miss reaching the laboratory confirmation, although blood culture sensitivity is around 60%. The culture-based diagnosis is ordinarily inaccessible in rural areas of poorly developed and developing countries. Even in urban areas, inadequate laboratory and diagnostic infrastructure in most tropical countries also contribute to the low reporting of cases.[1,2]

TRANSMISSION AND PREVENTION

There are no proven reports of spreading the causative bacterium from person to person. Hence, isolating the infected person may not be appropriate for preventing melioidosis. It is essential to target the risk factors. Some important public health strategies are described later in the chapter.

TRANSMISSION THROUGH SOIL AND WATER

The infection is known to be acquired when damaged skin comes in contact with contaminated mud or water.[4] Modes of transmission and their preventions are shown in

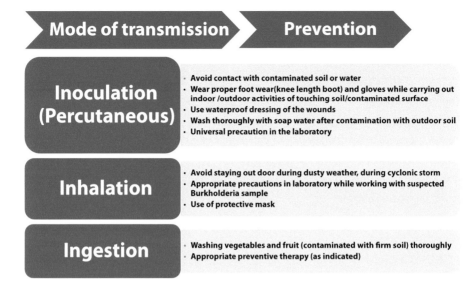

FIGURE 17.1   Mode of transmission and methods of prevention of melioidosis.

Figure 17.1. The organism is known to remain in the soil adjacent to the roots of plants and the surface groundwater of tropical and sub-tropical areas.[2,5]

Protective gloves must be worn to prevent cutaneous spread when working with loose soil and mud, where the bacteria survive. During the rainy season, farmers working in watery fields in mud, i.e., rice fields, must use water-resistant 'knee-high' boots.[6] One must restrict routine and recreational activities without barrier protections involving soil handling, such as gardening and agriculture. Similarly, one must avoid water contamination by avoiding swimming or fishing in rivers, lakes, or ponds. In Northern Australia, periodic basic health education is usually given to such occupational groups and the target population to prevent contamination directly from the soil and water.[6]

In a study, nearly 97% of the rice-farming and rural population were unaware of the disease transmission.[4] The inherent tradition of habits, discomfort, and economic constraints are the barriers to not wearing protective footwear and accepting the change.[4]

The tropical climate of the coastal areas in the tropical region, having increased rainfall and temperature, loose soil, paddy cultivation, and unprotected workers in civil construction, are strongly favourable for melioidosis.[7] A population with a high prevalence of diabetes is more susceptible. In highly endemic areas, the transmission of melioidosis occurs in humans by the inhalation of dust contaminated with organisms embedded in soil particles in the form of aerosols.[8] There is a need to remind people not to go out during storms in tropical climates.

PREVENTION OF WATER CONTAMINATION

A survey in Australia revealed that 33% of groundwater (borewell water) was contaminated with *B. pseudomallei*. Ultraviolet irradiation effectively disinfected the untreated

TABLE 17.1   Modifiable risk factors[12–20]

MODIFIABLE RISK FACTORS FOR MELIOIDOSIS
Diabetes mellitus
Prolonged glucocorticoid use
Immunosuppression
Heavy alcohol use
Barefoot exposure to soil (particularly in the rainy season)
Outdoor exposure to stormy or cyclonic weather
Smoking
Chronic pulmonary disease
Chronic renal disease
Chronic liver disease
Hemoglobinopathies
Occupational exposures
Chronic heart diseases
Human Immunodeficiency Virus infection/AIDS
Systemic lupus erythematous (SLE)

bore water supplies in a subsequent study.[9,10] Large-scale chlorination has shown to be a useful way to disinfect potable water to control melioidosis in Australia.[11] In places where the use of ultraviolet light for water treatment is not feasible, boiling water is a viable option for safe drinking water.[9]

PREVENTION OF RISK FACTORS

Prevention of the emergence of risk factors (primordial prevention) in the development of melioidosis (Table 17.1), such as diabetes, chronic airways, and parenchymal lung disease, chronic renal disease, heavy alcoholism, and heavy smoking, are important.[12,13] Important modifiable risk factors for melioidosis are listed in the Table 17.1.

OTHER EXPERIMENTAL MODALITIES

Early diagnosis and appropriate antibiotic treatment decreases morbidity and mortality and should stop the further spread of infection. *B. pseudomallei* has the tremendous capacity to persist in the soil and environment, even in adverse conditions, which is a constraint for prevention. Chitosan, a non-toxic polysaccharide biopolymer, impedes *Burkholderia's* growth and causes cell death by extracellular release of its intracellular content.[21] Calcium oxide is known to have bactericidal activity by *in vitro* study, decreasing the risk of infection from contaminated paddy field soil.[21] Similar preventive soil management with calcium oxide was proven beneficial in a Thai zoo in environmental control.[22]

PUBLIC HEALTH AWARENESS CAMPAIGN

The utilization of modern-day social media and the promotion of various preventive approaches must be encouraged. Those approaches are protective footwear and water chlorination, particularly for those at high-risk, are to be encouraged.

The universal approach of information, education, and communication activities in the community motivates people to take preventive steps as far as possible. Health education in public places and schools increases health awareness.

Various steps in the prevention and control approach by the World Health Organization (WHO) for neglected tropical diseases (NTDs) are: (1) preventive chemotherapy, (2) intensified case management, (3) control of disease vectors, (4) provision of clean water and sanitation, and (5) veterinary public health measures. These multi-step approaches can improve long-term infection prevention.[23]

PREVENTION OF INFECTION IN HEALTHCARE SETTINGS

The hazard for transmission of *B. pseudomallei* in a laboratory setup is usually low. Laboratory staff must reduce their risk of exposure through good laboratory practices. The laboratory staff needs training to adopt universal precautions and good laboratory practices to handle the organism under a biosafety level 3 (BSL-3) condition.[24] Wherever feasible, BSL-3 facilities are ideal but may not be feasible in all the laboratories where the disease is endemic.

POST-EXPOSURE PROPHYLAXIS (PEP)

There is a very negligible risk from laboratory contamination. The contamination of the bacteria through penetration of skin injuries, mouth, or eyes, and accidental exposure to the aerosols near or outside of a biosafety cabinet has substantial theoretical risks.[25] The risk assessment must be done after each exposure episode for post-exposure prophylaxis (PEP). The standard PEP is oral trimethoprim-sulfamethoxazole (cotrimoxazole), doxycycline, or co-amoxiclav may be given for 21 days.[25] The potential benefit of PEP must be weighed against the adverse effect of trimethoprim-sulfamethoxazole, mainly when there are low-risk exposures. The risk factors like uncontrolled diabetes and definite exposure can be an indication of PEP.[26]

DEVELOPMENT OF VACCINES

There is no licensed vaccine available at present. One vaccine using outer membrane vesicles (OMV) of *B. pseudomallei* has been found to be highly immunogenic. The immunization of mice with enhanced OMV showed significant protection against pulmonary infection.[27] Only one vaccine has been launched for human trials (phase 1 clinical trial). So far, a single study on vaccination has been published from Northeast Thailand to find possible cost-effectiveness.[28] Until a suitable vaccine is approved for human use, prevention remains the key strategy.

Live attenuated vaccines induce good immune responses by eliciting both humoral and cellular immunity in a mouse model. This vaccine for melioidosis has the potential to protect particularly against inhalational melioidosis.[29] An *in vitro* model by priming human T cells with dendritic cells is being developed, which can assess components of *B. pseudomallei* and has utility in developing subunit vaccines.[30]

Melioidosis surveillance: Since rice farming while barefoot is common in suburban and rural areas in many tropical countries, surveillance in such areas should initially focus on estimating the burden of the disease, detecting disease outbreaks, and characterizing persons with greater risk for diseases.

CONCLUSION

Primordial prevention by stopping the emergence of risk factors and a multi-modal approach to the prevention of melioidosis is possibly the best way to control transmission and the disease. Primary public health preventive measures like good hygiene, the use of barrier methods like water-resistant 'knee-high' boots and hand gloves, safe drinking water, and restriction of outdoor movement during dusty storms and cyclones are the keys to preventing melioidosis. The impact of the disease can be further decreased by establishing awareness of its endemicity by officially recognizing melioidosis as a neglected tropical disease.[31]

REFERENCES

1. Birnie E, et al. Global Burden of Melioidosis in 2015: A Systematic Review and Data Synthesis. Lancet Infect Dis 2019; 19(8): 892–902.
2. Limmathurotsakul D, et al. Predicted Global Distribution of *Burkholderia pseudomallei* and Burden of Melioidosis. Nat Microbiol 2016; 1(1): 15008.

3. Chai LYA, et al. Earth, Wind, Rain, and Melioidosis. Lancet Planet Health 2018; 2(8): e329–e30.

4. Suntornsut P, et al. Barriers and Recommended Interventions to Prevent Melioidosis in Northeast Thailand: A Focus Group Study Using the Behaviour Change Wheel. PLoS Negl Trop Dis 2016; 10(7): e0004823.

5. Kaestli M, et al. Out of the Ground: Aerial and Exotic Habitats of the Melioidosis Bacterium *Burkholderia pseudomallei* in Grasses in Australia. Environ Microbiol 2012; 14(8): 2058–70.

6. Hinjoy S, et al. Melioidosis in Thailand: Present and Future. Trop Med Infect Dis 2018; 3(2): 38.

7. Behera B, et al. Melioidosis in Odisha: A Clinico-Microbiological and Epidemiological Description of Culture-Confirmed Cases Over a 2-Year Period. Indian J Med Microbiol 2019; 37(3): 430–32.

8. Chen PS, et al. Airborne Transmission of Melioidosis to Humans from Environmental Aerosols Contaminated with *B. pseudomallei*. PLoS Negl Trop Dis 2015; 9(6): e0003834.

9. McRobb E, et al. Melioidosis from Contaminated Bore Water and Successful UV Sterilization. Am J Trop Med Hyg 2013; 89(2): 367–8.

10. Mayo M, et al. *Burkholderia pseudomallei* in Unchlorinated Domestic Bore Water, Tropical Northern Australia. Emerg Infect Dis 2011; 17(7): 1283–5.

11. Howard K, et al. Disinfection of *Burkholderia pseudomallei* in Potable Water. Water Res 2005; 39(6): 1085–92.

12. Sridharan S, et al. Melioidosis in Critical Care: A Review. Indian J Crit Care Med 2021; 25(Suppl 2): S161–S65.

13. Meumann EM, et al. Clinical Features and Epidemiology of Melioidosis Pneumonia: Results from a 21-Year Study and Review of the Literature. Clin Infect Dis 2012; 54(3): 362–9.

14. Limmathurotsakul D, et al. Increasing Incidence of Human Melioidosis in Northeast Thailand. Am J Trop Med Hyg 2010; 82(6): 1113–7.

15. Currie BJ, et al. The Epidemiology and Clinical Spectrum of Melioidosis: 540 Cases from the 20 Year Darwin Prospective Study. PLoS Negl Trop Dis 2010; 4(11): e900.

16. Currie BJ, et al. Melioidosis Epidemiology and Risk Factors from a Prospective Whole-Population Study in Northern Australia. Trop Med Int Health 2004; 9(11): 1167–74.

17. Fong SM, et al. Thalassemia Major is a Major Risk Factor for Pediatric Melioidosis in Kota Kinabalu, Sabah, Malaysia. Clin Infect Dis 2015; 60(12): 1802–7.

18. Kronsteiner B, et al. Diabetes Alters Immune Response Patterns to Acute Melioidosis in Humans. Eur J Immunol 2019; 49(7): 1092–106.

19. Wiersinga WJ, et al. Melioidosis. Nat Rev Dis Primers 2018; 4: 17107.

20. Menon R, et al. Risk Factors for Mortality in Melioidosis: A Single-Centre, 10-Year Retrospective Cohort Study. Sci. World J 2021; 2021: 8154810.

21. Kamjumphol W, et al. Antibacterial Activity of Chitosan Against *Burkholderia pseudomallei*. Microbiologyopen 2018; 7(1): e00534.

22. Sommanustweechai A, et al. Environmental Management Procedures Following Fatal Melioidosis in a Captive Chimpanzee (Pan troglodytes). J Zoo Wildl Med 2013; 44(2): 475–9.

23. Mohapatra PR, et al. Melioidosis. Lancet Infect Dis 2019; 19(10): 1056–57.

24. Peacock SJ, et al. Management of Accidental Laboratory Exposure to *Burkholderia pseudomallei* and B. mallei. Emerg Infect Dis 2008; 14(7): e2.

25. Lipsitz R, et al. Workshop on Treatment of and Postexposure Prophylaxis for *Burkholderia pseudomallei* and *B. mallei* Infection, 2010. Emerg Infect Dis 2012; 18(12): e2.

26. Dance DA, et al. *Burkholderia pseudomallei*: Challenges for the Clinical Microbiology Laboratory-a Response from the Front Line. J Clin Microbiol 2017; 55(3): 980–82.

27. Grund ME, et al. Thinking Outside the Bug: Targeting Outer Membrane Proteins for *Burkholderia* Vaccines. Cells 2021; 10(3): 495.

28. Peacock SJ, et al. Melioidosis Vaccines: A Systematic Review and Appraisal of the Potential to Exploit Biodefense Vaccines for Public Health Purposes. PLoS Negl Trop Dis 2012; 6(1): e1488.
29. Khakhum N, et al. Antigen-Specific Antibody and Polyfunctional T Cells Generated by Respiratory Immunization with Protective *Burkholderia* ΔtonB Δhcp1 Live Attenuated Vaccines. NPJ Vaccines 2021; 6(1): 72.
30. Reddi D, et al. *In Vitro* Priming of Human T Cells by Dendritic Cells Provides a Screening Tool for Candidate Vaccines for *Burkholderia pseudomallei*. Vaccines (Basel) 2021; 9(8): 929.
31. Savelkoel J, et al. A Call to Action: Time to Recognise Melioidosis as a Neglected Tropical Disease. Lancet Infect Dis 2021; 22(6): e176–82.

Index

Note: Locators in *italics* represent figures and **bold** indicate tables in the text.